The Gift of Life

—A MESSAGE OF HOPE FOR THE SERIOUSLY ILL

The Gift of Life

—A MESSAGE OF HOPE FOR THE SERIOUSLY ILL

Randy Becton

QUALITY PUBLICATIONS
P.O. BOX 1060 ABILENE, TEXAS 79604

formerly titled *We're All Terminal*

The author's proceeds from this book support the CARING cancer ministry.

Cover photograph by F. Miles Ezell, Jr.
Inside photographs by David Dillard

ISBN: 0-89137-309-8
formerly 0-89137-308-X

To Landon Saunders

Preface

The Gift of Life was written during the first year following the discovery that I had cancer. That diagnosis came in November 1973. As I write this preface in September 1978, it has been almost five years since this crisis began. It has been difficult. It has, however, been a blessing. My physical health at present is stable. I have recently celebrated my twelfth anniversary; we have just completed the adoption of our fourth child. Praise be to God for His goodness!

In the time since I first recorded the thoughts in this book, God has helped me to grow spiritually. Some of the ideas in this book have become more deeply ingrained in me, having more meaning with each new day. Some of the feelings and observations mellowed, changing slightly as I gained more perspective. A few thoughts have been abandoned as faulty or not useful, though at the time they were real.

Still, I have decided to share the material much as it was when I first wrote it. Otherwise it would not be what it was meant to be: a spiritual diary of thoughts and feelings during my first year with cancer.

In any case, much of what is here is still valid after five years. Life remains uncertain, a gift of God. Though everyone is terminal, Christians are eternal through our response to God's grace. Every sunrise is still a message from God. God is my Father.

I pray that what is here may speak to you in some way. If there is anything here that causes you to use a day a little better, or even to alter your life's direction and priorities in some way, I will thank God that the book has served some purpose.

Table of Contents

Foreword

The struggle to believe is possibly the mightiest conflict known to the soul of man. Faith does not always come from quiet contemplation or meditation. It is sometimes born among the raging of questions with no answers, pain with no relief, hope that has no reason to exist. It may be true that still waters run deep but only the restless ocean can bring the glistening sand of the peaceful seashore.

I have known Randy Becton for more than a decade. We have shared intimacies, dreams, doubts and disasters. We have been foolish and lighthearted; somber and dejected. I know the man.

"It hurts and I'm worried" he said as he told me of recurring pains and achings. Neither of us realized that surgery would reveal not only a devastating illness but predict a long season of suffering both in soul and body. There would soon be literally dozens of tests, hundred of injections and a thousand times of asking "why?" There would soon be a struggle, not only to survive, but to believe. It would not be a light skirmish with whether or not God created the universe. It would be a full-scale battle against the devil in the hell of doubt and pain.

The devil lost. Randy survived physically and spiritually. His faith and experience have led him to open his life to those who read this book. His better look at what is real, and even more essential, what is important, is the product of the stark reality of facing death and reflecting all of life's activities and loyalties against that dark screen.

Experience is always the teacher. We sometimes do not learn from it but I know that Randy has learned and has, through this book, shared that learning with us. I sincerely recommend it to you as an aid in the struggle to believe, to *really* believe.

Glenn Owen
September 1978

The Gift of Life

—A MESSAGE OF HOPE FOR THE SERIOUSLY ILL

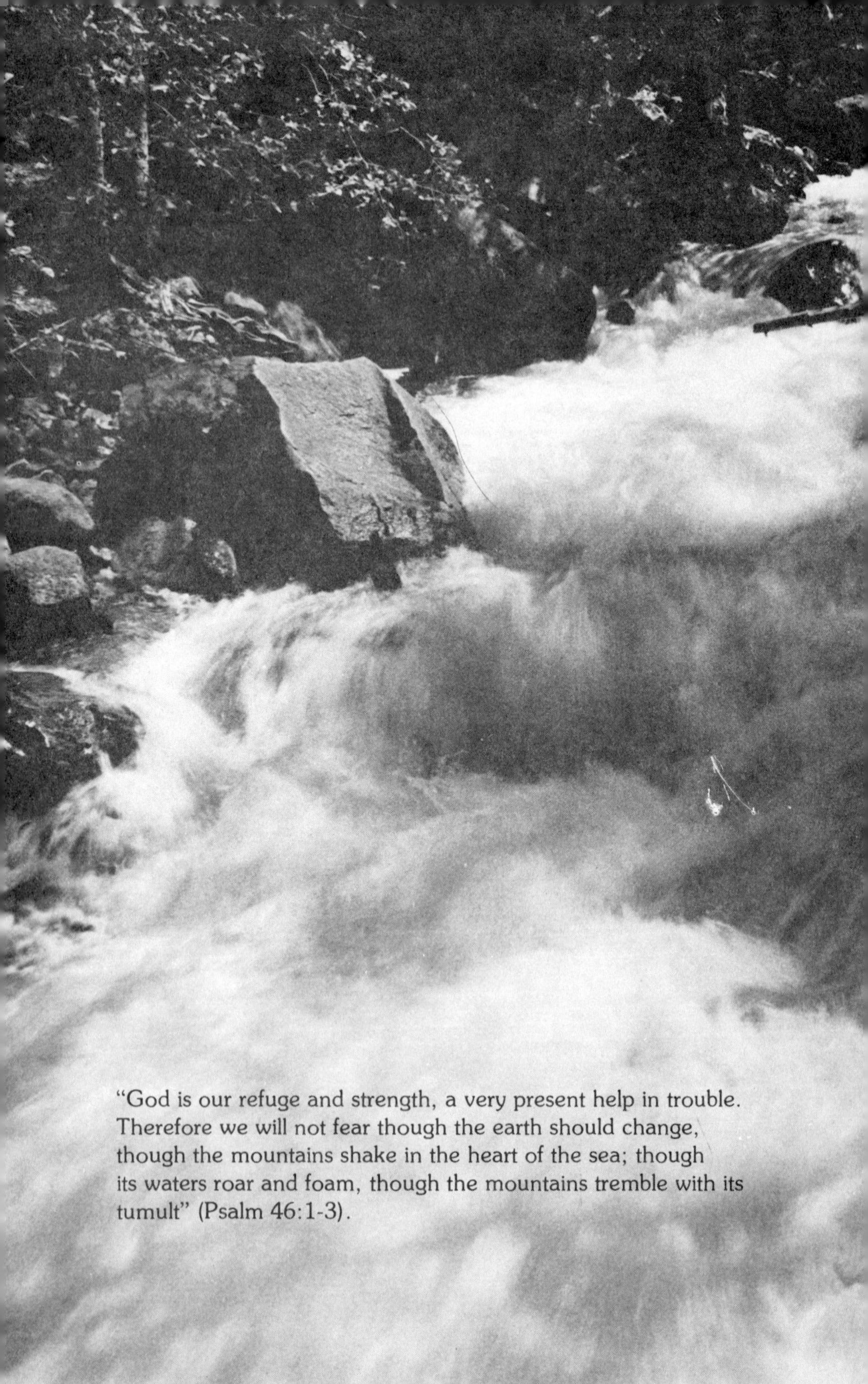

"God is our refuge and strength, a very present help in trouble. Therefore we will not fear though the earth should change, though the mountains shake in the heart of the sea; though its waters roar and foam, though the mountains tremble with its tumult" (Psalm 46:1-3).

A Search for Understanding

Why am I writing this? I've asked myself that question quite a few times. There are several reasons. Perhaps primary is my belief that each one of us will experience a crisis in his life at some time. It may be a crisis of health, occupation, emotional stress or any of a number of things. How do you respond to a crisis? Although I do not offer set formulas, I do feel that the experiences of others help us to soberly think through and evaluate our own experiences. Maybe we can develop a sense of perspective. My health crisis has profoundly changed my life. I've been given several opportunities to share with groups and individuals some of the changes in my thinking. By writing down some of these reflections I hope to make them available to those whom my life touches as well as some whom I may never meet.

Another reason for writing down reflections is to continually evaluate the worth of my own thoughts. Are they valid? Do they square with the way things really are? Are they honest? Are they consistent with God's revealed truths? I've decided that one way to find these answers and others is to put the thoughts down on paper.

Finally, I have a deep belief that I have been granted life for a specific reason. Although it may be difficult to understand, I think God has spared my life so that through these experiences some people may be led to consider God's place in their lives. I treasure the possibility that my life might be used by God to draw people closer to Him. When Jesus, in John 11, heard of the sickness of his dear friend, Lazarus, he said,

> The purpose of his illness is not death, but for the glory of God.

I have prayed, from the earliest days in the hospital in Houston, that this could be true of my life. I am well aware that God can be glorified by death as well as by life. Yet it was and still is my hope that through His healing work my life might be a living testimony to the fact that He lives, He loves, and He is active on behalf of men. As I have said to several groups already, even if my health fails in the near future I am convinced that these last few months have demonstrated His goodness in my life. Hopefully the following pages will show what God has done.

If sharing these thoughts helps to move even one person one step closer to God our Father, I will feel richly rewarded. If you wish more (or less) had been developed on a given subject, please understand that I really did not intend to say the final word on anything. I prefer that you develop these thoughts more fully on your own; it will be enough if they stimulate your thinking.

In talking with individuals or groups in college gatherings, Bible classes, worship services, retreat situations and other settings, I found that my thinking was best stimulated and most sharply focused by considering questions which people asked. However, almost all of these lines were written out of another setting: insomnia. One of my drugs has insomnia as its side effect, so many of these pages were written between 1 a.m. and 6 in the morning. I don't know whether that's significant or not!

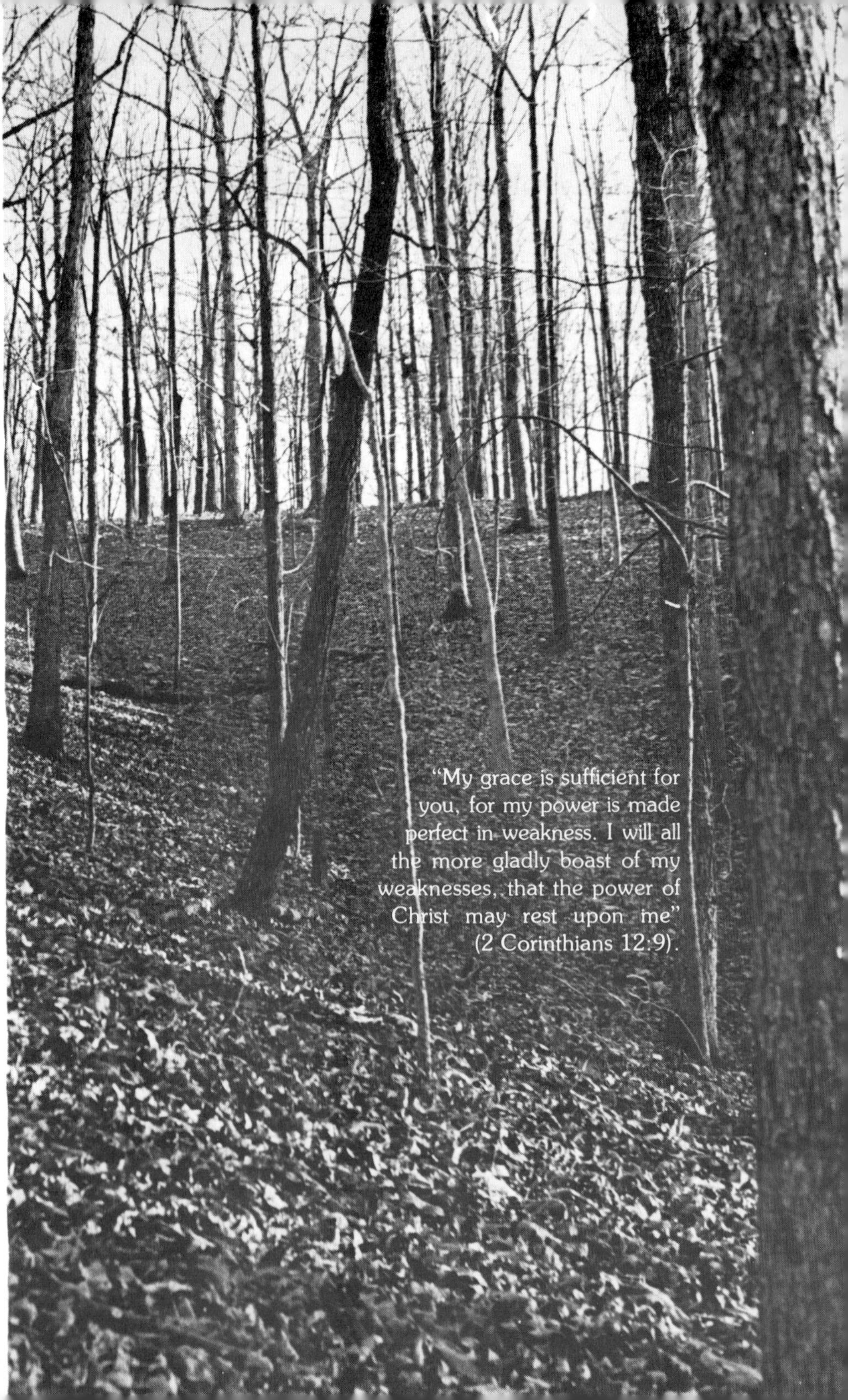
"My grace is sufficient for you, for my power is made perfect in weakness. I will all the more gladly boast of my weaknesses, that the power of Christ may rest upon me" (2 Corinthians 12:9).

The Medical Story Briefly

It began in October, 1973. A swollen stomach and general fatigue were the only symptoms during a week home from work. After antibiotics failed to alleviate the symptoms my doctor decided to admit me to West Texas Hospital for tests to seek the source of the problem. After x-rays and tests of various kinds, the results of the lab reports revealed Lymphosarcoma, cancer of the lymph system. Hearing the result of the diagnosis was a terrible shock. (It is an experience that more than one-half million Americans will have this year.)

After undergoing abdominal surgery to determine the extent and exact nature of the cancer, preparations were immediately made for me to be sent to M. D. Anderson Hospital and Tumor Institute in Houston, Texas. After a total of ten days in West Texas Hospital, I was flown by private plane to Houston, where I was admitted. An excellent team of doctors began to determine which course of treatment held the most promise for my type of cancer. Through further tests and study of the biopsy reports, the doctors, using computerized information, decided upon a program of treatment using chemotherapy. Since the cancer had already affected the kidneys and lungs by the time I arrived in Houston, I was extremely ill during those first days. On the fourth day, the staff came in and began the chemotherapy treatment. There were four drugs: Adriamycin, Cytoxan, Vincristne and Prednisone. The first three were given intravenously, the last orally. My physical system was badly jolted by these powerful drugs; the drug reaction lasted about three days and nights. These reactions to the chemotherapy treatments were probably the hardest part of my hospitalization. Fortunately my body adjusted gradually to them and they became easier to take each time. During the three weeks in M. D. Anderson, I received three rounds of chemotherapy. Gradually, I began to feel better until finally I was released to continue chemotherapy as an outpatient of the hospital.

Since being released from the hospital, I have been continuing chemotherapy. From November to June, I received treatments every third week. I reported regularly for check-ups in Houston. My visit in June was thrilling, for I was told that the cancer had gone into total remission. Remission means that the cancer is totally inactive at present. This is the goal of chemotherapy since at this point there is no cure for Lymphosarcoma. The first rounds of chemotherapy are referred to as "inductive," designed to stop the growth of the cancer, while the later treatments are called "maintenance" treatments and are designed to maintain remission.

There have been a few problems caused by the chemotherapy. The principal problem was an intestinal obstruction which was quite painful for several months until major surgery corrected it. Shortly after this surgery, an abdominal abscess appeared. Chemotherapy causes the white blood cell count to dip to a low number, resulting in susceptibility to infection. Surgery also corrected the abscess. Further side affects occurred but were not too serious.

At the time of this writing, the chemotherapy treatment continues with Cytoxan and Prednisone, at 16-day intervals for five consecutive days at each treatment. Periodic check-ups continue. The chemotherapy will be continued for approximately 15 more months if the cancer remains in remission. What are the long-term possibilities of life? No one can say. It is hoped that I can be a long-term survivor.

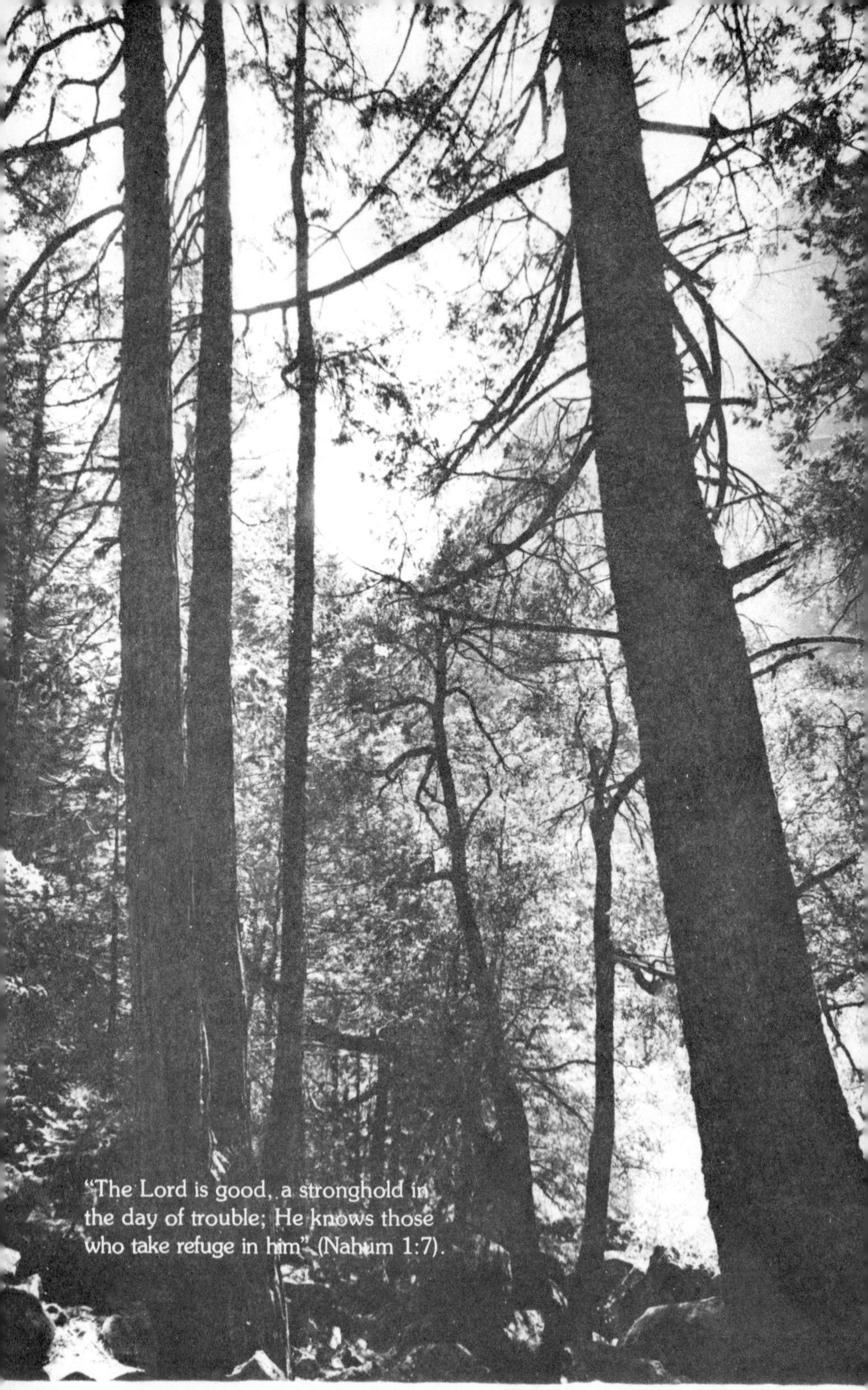
"The Lord is good, a stronghold in the day of trouble; He knows those who take refuge in him" (Nahum 1:7).

God as Father

One of the difficult things in life is to find an adequate view of God. Although God is described in many ways in the Bible, I believe each person must come to his own perception of God's real nature and of what relationship He actually has to our life. In a serious crisis, such as I experienced, one searches even more frantically for a helpful concept of God. At least, I did.

I've always been fascinated by the contemplation of what a perfect father would be like. Even though most of us would say there is no "ideal" human father, there is no one with whom I've talked on the subject who cannot imagine what he would envision an ideal father to be. Everyone can tell you something about his "ideal father."

In Houston, this thought repeatedly found a place in my thinking. I had heard God described as the Great Creator and Sustainer of the Universe, as the Mighty God, and as many other things. Yet I needed to experience God's presence and love for me in a personal rather than an abstract way. That's why the thought of God as my heavenly Father became so special to me. How helpless I felt! How alone! In fact, the strongest single emotion that I experienced was the loneliness caused by suffering and the uncertainty of facing the unknown.

CRYING OUT TO THE FATHER

I do not know of anything in this whole world that is worse than this feeling of being alone. I needed a loving Father who would surround me with His understanding, His arms of love. I felt like Jesus must have felt when he went into the Garden of Gethsemane, taking his disciples with him to pray. In Mark 14, verse 32, the scripture reports that he told them, "My soul is very sorrowful, even to death . . ." and verse 36 says,

> And he said, "Abba, Father, all things are possible to thee; remove this cup from me; yet not what I will, but what thou wilt."

Jesus uses the intimate, personal "Abba" in speaking to his Father about the deepest concern of his heart. The hour was near, the weight of all the world's sin was heavy upon him, the fact of his death was imminent, and Jesus shared his burden of anxiety with God by asking that the cup be removed.

His example inspired me to feel that my deepest feelings were safe with God. I was convinced that it is right to cry out to God. It is an appropriate response of our humanity to bare ourselves before Him in the midst of our suffering, our pain, our disappointments, as well as our hopes, expectations and joys. I believe it is always proper for a child to be honest with his father, and to ask anything from his father; but also helpful to me was Jesus' ready submission to the Father's will.

While it is proper to express our will to God fully, it must follow that our spirit acknowledges the Father's ultimately superior wisdom and ways. I prayed for the gift of life; I asked God, repeatedly, to allow me to live. I told Him all my reasons for so desiring, knowing that He fully understood each of them. He knows a father's yearning for his young children to know him and his longing to be present during their formative years. He knows the depth of a man's love for his wife. He knows the zest for life and the love of life that men hold precious. He identifies with the motives of one who wishes to see more fruit from his life's work. Still, after acknowledging all this, Jesus suggests that God knows what's best for His children. I've become convinced that man's eyesight is limited—he only sees "as through a glass darkly." He tends to seek to direct his own footsteps instead of heeding the wise admonition:

> Trust in the Lord with all your heart and do not rely on your own insight, In all your ways acknowledge him; and he will make straight your paths (Proverbs 3:5,6).

Paul wrote to Christians at Rome about God as their Father, referring to the spirit of sonship:

> For you did not receive the spirit of slavery to fall back into fear, but you have received the spirit of sonship. When we cry, "Abba! Father!" it is the Spirit himself bearing witness with our spirit that we are children of God, and if children, then heirs, heirs of God and fellow heirs with Christ . . . (Romans 8:15-17).

Do you mean that I, like Jesus, can intimately call on God, "Abba Father"? Definitely, if I am His son. When I responded to Jesus Christ as Saviour and Lord through baptism, I became a child of God.

John 1:12 says that to those who received him, "he gave power to become children of God. . . ."

In Romans 8:18-25, Paul goes on to say that although decay and death characterize this earthly life, the children of God, as well as creation itself, all look forward to God's ultimate action: "the redemption of our bodies." How reassuring it is to know what the Father plans for His children.

Paul tells the Ephesian Christians that "He (God) destined us in love to be His sons through Jesus Christ" (Ephesians 1:5). To the Galatians he wrote:

> But when the time had fully come, God sent forth his Son, born of woman, born under the law, to redeem those who were under the law, so that we might receive adoption as sons. And because you are sons, God has sent the Spirit of his Son into our hearts, crying "Abba! Father!" So through God you are no longer a slave but a son, and if a son then an heir (Galatians 4:4-7).

A SON TRUSTS

What did all this mean to me? I am God's son. What an honor! He has adopted me into His family. He is willing to be my loving Heavenly Father. Oh, if we could only begin to see the promise, the security, the joy and the future that is real and certain because God is our Father. I know this—I know my Father, I trust my Father and I love my Father. "Abba, Father." This sustained me through serious sickness, and is an anchor point in my life at this moment. A letter I received when I was hospitalized reminded me of a real truth: "We need never fear the next moment when we know we possess the last hour." When I think that my Father lovingly controls the last hour, then trusting Him with the next moment is not so difficult. I remember too that my Father said:

> I want you to trust me in your times of trouble, so I can rescue you, and you can give me glory (Psalm 50:15 LB).

"For none of us lives to himself alone and none of us dies to himself alone. If we live, we live to the Lord, and if we die, we die to the Lord. So, whether we live or die, we belong to the Lord" (Romans 14:7,8).

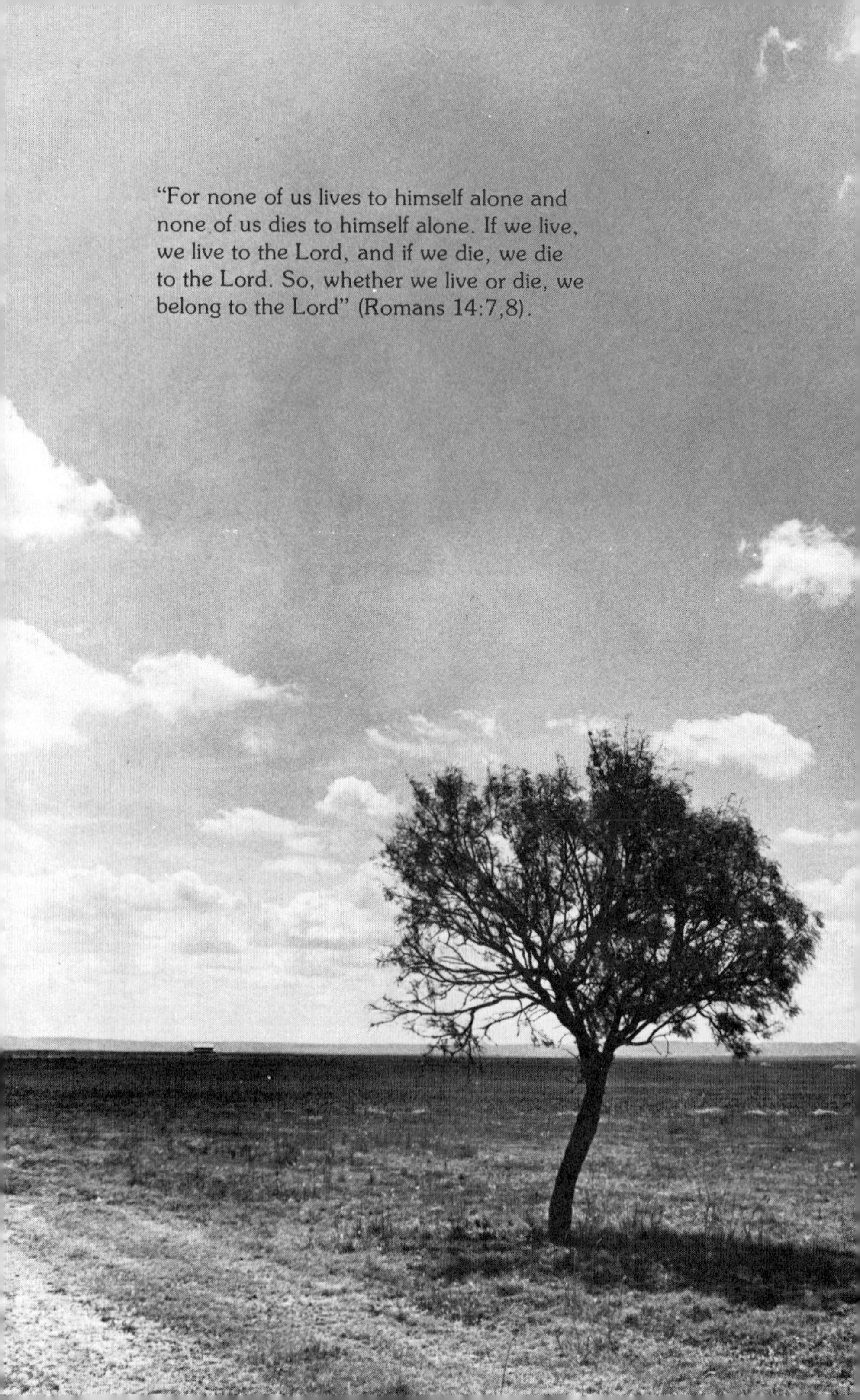

Everyone is Terminal

The bright young interviewer from the newspaper sat in my office asking me to reflect on my adjustments to the reality of cancer. Her primary interest was to learn if I could cope with this sorrowful fact. During our 2½-hour visit, at one point I said, "Well, when you think about it, we are all terminal." Her response indicated that she had never thought about death in this way. In fact, so struck was she that she entitled the article, "The Thing Is Everyone Is Terminal."

I first thought of that phrase when reading an encouraging letter from a missionary couple in Guatemala. They told me that several couples had gathered for a devotional and had prayed specifically for me. One veteran missionary in the group prayed, "Lord help us to remember that we are all terminal." How true it is. None will escape the death experience.

A friend of mine once commented on the fact that of all the philosophies of life written by the various philosophers down through time, none of them had adequately coped with the problem of death. Death mystifies us, doesn't it? Most of us are horribly afraid of it. It stands against everything we are for. We view it as our personal enemy.

TOO CLOSE TO DEATH

You may wonder how my health experience has affected my view toward death; needless to say, I have thought about death often in this illness. It is certainly a very near possibility for me. In fact, during the three weeks in Houston, I doubted that I would recover. Many times I felt I would not see home again. Even when released I fought against the feeling that I was being released in order to come home to die. How close I actually was to death, I don't know, but I felt very close. I don't know how close I am now, but one thing is certain—at some point I will die and you will die. There is nothing profitable in refusing to face this truth. There is much profit in allowing this truth to give you insight into the meaning of your life. The Psalmist says:

> So teach us to number our days that we may get a heart of wisdom (Psalm 90:12).

One time a friend said to me that he felt a man was not equipped to live until he was prepared to die. Is there truth in that?

My experience in facing death may or may not be helpful to you. I cannot say what all men experience, only what I experienced at this time. First of all, I viewed death as a horrible enemy, not as a friend. Life snuffed out by cancer at 29? Disease triumphant over life? How could one in my position welcome that prospect? No, death wouldn't come as a friend at all. Now I am aware that the Apostle Paul told the Philippians that to depart and be with the Lord would be "far better" (Philippians 1:23) and that "to live is Christ and to die is gain" (Philippians 1:21). I also recall the verse which says "precious in the sight of the Lord is the death of his saints" (Psalm 116:15). Paul's stance is admirable, commendable, and beautiful—but right now in my life it is simply not my stance. I am trying to make progress toward this view, but my desire to live on earth is very strong at this time. I pray that God's will is to grant me life. However, I also pray that if His will is death, I may meet that with living faith and glorify Him through it. Still, I do not believe that we are asked to be indifferent about death.

What about the fear of death? No doubt, I was afraid. There are still periods of fear. Whether it's the fear of the unknown or the fear of something else I don't know. I just know it's there, and furthermore I feel that it is normal.

SOURCES OF COMFORT

I am assisted in overcoming fear by God's promise of His presence.

> Yea though I walk through the valley of the shadow of death I will fear no evil for thou art with me . . . (Psalm 23:4).

I am also helped by Jesus' assertion:

> I am the resurrection and the life; he who believes in me, though he die, yet shall he live, and whoever lives and believes in me shall never die (John 11:25,26).

I have no doubt that God will certainly keep His promise to raise me because I am in Jesus Christ:

> If the Spirit of him who raised Jesus from the dead dwells in you, he who raised Christ Jesus from the dead will give life to your mortal

> bodies also through his Spirit which dwells in you (Romans 8:11).
>
> But our commonwealth is in heaven, and from it we await a Savior, the Lord Jesus Christ, who will change our lowly body to be like his glorious body, by the power which enables him even to subject all things to himself (Philippians 3:20,21).

These passages and others help equip me to trust God in the death experience, but they do not ease all apprehension about that profound event. When I speak on this subject it sometimes shocks people that I admit fears and apprehensions. Maybe it's because some feel that there is no place in a life of faith for fear. All I can say is that in confronting the fear of death with the power of faith, that faith became more meaningful to me. Still, that confrontation is a lifelong struggle. Maybe some of us make more progress than others. I notice progress in my life through this experience, but if you ask me if the battle is over I will honestly tell you, "No!"

I can't begin to tell you how encouraging and how meaningful to me personally the following thought is: one of the reasons Jesus took human nature upon himself was

> He himself likewise partook of the same nature, that through death he might destroy him who has the power of death, that is, the devil, and deliver all those who through fear of death were subject to lifelong bondage (Hebrews 2:14,15).

What a blessing! Man's enemy rendered powerless by my Lord Jesus Christ. That is why I know I will be victorious over fear, for indeed, there now is nothing real to fear. (You see, I told you I am making progress.) Jesus "tasted death for every one" (Hebrews 2:9), therefore I am a participant in eternal life which is his gift:

> The wages of sin is death, but the free gift of God is eternal life in Christ Jesus our Lord (Romans 6:23).

Yes, everyone is terminal because sin brought death into this world (Romans 5:12), but Jesus brought life (Romans 5:18). In a relationship with Him I live and you live. That's why I am thrilled and drawn toward that final day when

> the perishable puts on the imperishable, and the mortal puts on immortality, then shall come to pass the saying that is written: "Death is swallowed up in victory" (1 Corinthians 15:54).

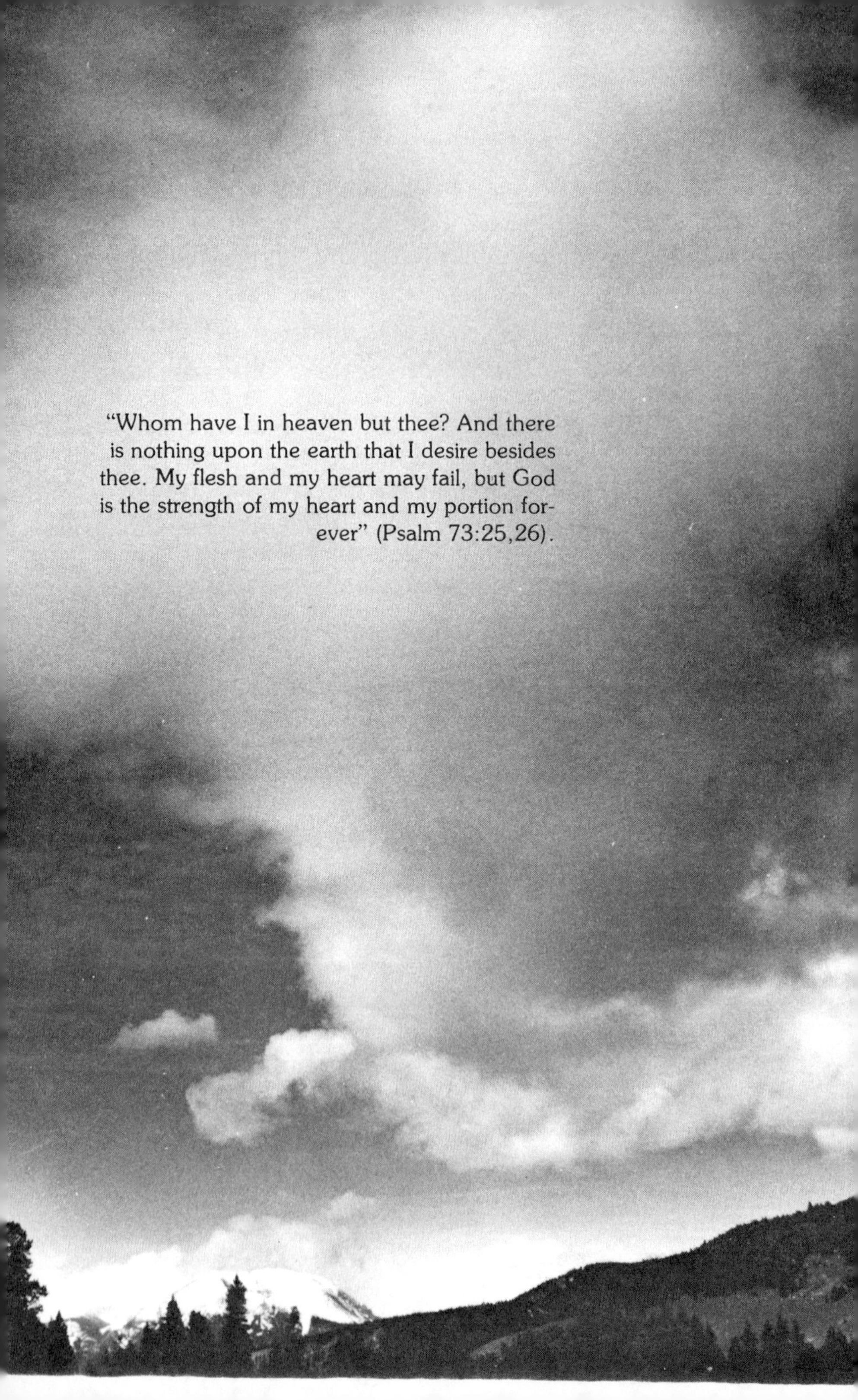

"Whom have I in heaven but thee? And there is nothing upon the earth that I desire besides thee. My flesh and my heart may fail, but God is the strength of my heart and my portion forever" (Psalm 73:25,26).

The Network of Concern

During these last twelve months I have received many expressions of love and concern in the form of cards and letters. These contributed significantly to my spiritual and emotional health, as well as encouraging me in the battle to regain physical health. Many cards came from Christians who simply but beautifully let me know that they cared and that my situation was constantly receiving attention in their prayers. Although some of the expressions were intensely personal, I feel that sharing some of these with you may be profitable. Maybe in some of these expressions you will find models for ministering to people through cards and letters. More than this, however, I hope that you may see the depth of faith and hope that these individuals share in order to encourage and sustain me in their "network of concern."

Obviously, I could not include all that were received, nor do I want to leave the impression that these were the most helpful. I received each at different points along the way in the struggle and each spoke to me in its own way from the life of someone who really cared. All were blessings. All of the following excerpts are from people whom I know and who know me.

Early in my illness a dear Christian missionary couple in Zambia wrote:

> May God enfold you in His great love and lift you up from all pain and sorrow. We wish so much to talk to you face to face, but pray that you will feel our love stretching out over all these miles. We believe in God's power above everything else and that He is in control of your lives as well as ours. If we could only see as He does!

A Christian brother from Tennessee wrote perceptively:

> I don't fully grasp why you walk this valley but I fully trust the Lord who walks it with you and know that even this will bring glory to His name. We pray He'll lift you up. We know you'll lift Him up and we're excited that your life is used to draw needy men to our all-sufficient Christ.

In these months this brother's observation has proved true. Some lives have been drawn nearer. Different people have allowed our experience to cause them to re-evaluate their priorities and commitments. One brother said it this way:

> Your illness has brought us all closer together and to God, and it has helped me to re-evaluate my life. In three days I will be 30, and I have wondered if I could meet the great challenge to your faith that has faced you in these recent days . . . .

A letter from Indonesia reflected on my experience and concluded:

> I have about decided that to live in the certainty of Jesus Christ is to live in the utmost uncertainty as far as the world is concerned.

From California:

> You and your family have made us so rich in life . . . you have taught us so much . . . live each minute . . . each day.

A dear sister wrote:

> I often wonder how people make it sanely through times of stress who do not know the Lord.

Three letters, selected from several, indicate the intensity of concern and the desire to participate in the experience with Camilla and myself. A brother in Houston wrote:

> I know there is no possible way to fully share the agony and the victory you have been going through the past few months. Perhaps it helps to know, though, that our hearts have been with you, and that so many of us really wanted to share all you've suffered. You have not been alone, not so much because of us, but because of Him who chooses to call us friends and brothers. He who possesses the last hour never needs to fear the next minute.

Six precious couples joined together to say:

> We love you and Camilla and we're ready to sacrifice with you.

A former co-worker from California wrote:

> While I respect the importance of you and Randy having a limited number of people to deal with, I would be on my way to be with you today if I thought my presence would be of value. That readiness shall remain. Do not

> hesitate to let me know how I might help. Any resource I have is yours.

Involvement like this lifts the Spirit and really does participate in the situation. How grateful to God I am for those whose concern is so genuine!

Some showed their love by sharing poetry or scripture that had become especially meaningful in their lives, hoping that we could identify and be strengthened. From Accra, Ghana a missionary couple shared from their reading this verse:

> Two glad services are ours,
> Both the Master loves to bless:
> First we serve with all our powers,
> Then with all our feebleness,
> Nothing else the soul uplifts
> Save to serve Him night and day;
> Serve Him when He gives His gifts,
> Serve Him when He takes away.

A college student wrote reminding me of a class I had taught discussing Christ's agony in Gethsemane. She reminded me that I said, "In Christ's weakness, he saw God's strength move in." She said:

> I've remembered that and it has helped me over many rough spots. Now I pray that this same thought can return to you and bring peace. My husband and I are praying for you and yours daily that your trouble and recovery will be characterized by this beautiful belief.

A grade school student asked in such a sweet sensitive way:

> God sees the sparrows as they feed,
> And God sees the gulls as they fly
> across the sea.

If God sees the sparrow and the seagull
too,
Won't God, in your time of need see you?

A college professor in Missouri shared this:

Be still my soul: thy God doth undertake
To guide the Future as He has the past.
Thy hope, thy confidence let nothing shake;
All now mysterious shall be bright at last.
Be still my soul: the waves and winds still know
His voice who ruled them while he dwelt below.

A former classmate from Tennessee, who works with people in crisis, shared from the Phillip's translation of 2 Corinthians 4:7:

We are handicapped on all sides
But we are never frustrated;
We are puzzled,
But never in despair.
We are persecuted,
But we never have to stand it alone.
We may be knocked down
But we are never knocked out!

A dear brother shared one of his favorite Old Testament scriptures with me, while I was in the lowest spirits in Houston. I took his letter out from the drawer of the bedside table often when I was lonely and found great peace through contemplating this simply expressed faith:

But I trust in thee, O Lord,
I say, "Thou art my God."
My times are in thy hand (Psalms 31:14,15)

From Memphis a widow wrote having just been ministered to by this reading from Isaiah:

They who wait for the Lord shall renew their
strength
They shall mount up with wings like eagles,
They shall run and not be weary
They shall walk and not faint.

The letter from an old man, in shaky handwriting, refreshed my spirit. During the more than ten years in which we had been close, we often dreamed together of great possibilities in service to God and man. He has always been a profound influence on my life because of his pure heart and lovely faith. Having never flown before, he was prepared at any point to come personally to minister to me, even though from a great distance. His letter, in part, read:

> Bless your hearts, I love you . . . You will do your best to be calm—study to be quiet and relaxed. Why not ask the elders to anoint with oil and pray? I read in the Book about this . . . Is He not great? Are we not grateful to be brothers in Christ? We are on our way to live with God but not until He is ready to take us . . . May you both trust *HIM* and look to Him for strength and wisdom.

In reflecting on this last letter I thought of how often I had considered that he would be at home with God many years, perhaps, before I would. Now developments may have changed that. What if I were there to greet him when he arrived! Wouldn't that be something? He made me again realize that definitely "we are on our way" and there is such security to be found in the contemplation that our destination is certain. It reminds me of what is said about the men of faith such as Abel, Abraham, Noah and others:

> These men of faith I have mentioned died without ever receiving all that God had promised them; but they saw it all awaiting them on ahead and were glad, for they agreed that this earth was not their real home but that they were just strangers visiting down here. And quite obviously when they talked like that, they were looking forward to their real home in heaven.
>
> If they had wanted to, they could have gone back to the good things of this world. But they didn't want to. They were living for heaven. And now God is not ashamed to be called their God, for He has made an heavenly city for them (Hebrews 11:13-16).

From an older lady came this fresh reminder:

> Wish you could have seen God's world come alive this morning—but then God is God indoors too—and may you feel His presence around you your every waking moment . . .

Two letters were special because they came from people with serious health problems. A young man, whom I had played with as a boy, suffers from cancer and is also taking chemotherapy. A beautifully committed Christian, he wrote:

> I realize, from first hand experience, the pain and trouble you are enduring. I have thought of you often since hearing of your experience . . . I can only suggest, as you well know, that the Lord cares for those in his family and watches over them daily. Put your trust in Him as we will, anticipating your full and speedy recovery.

A teenage girl wrote:

> I was told you was taking treatments for cancer.

> Don't feel let down. I've had thirteen different operations . . . I've had so many operations nobody can tell me anything about operations. My prayers are with you all the way . . . I'm not very well some days . . . So you're not by yourself.

In a different vein I was encouraged by hearing from some very special people—people that I was privileged to lead to Jesus Christ as Saviour and Lord. When I took time to re-evaluate my life's efforts, I had difficulty remembering significant things I had done that were contributions to God's purposes. There were several times when my 29 years passed before me for review. The review left me unsatisfied with many aspects of my past, as one might expect. However, a young woman in Kentucky and a middle-aged man in Tennessee brought real joy and thanksgiving. A part of her note read:

> I know you may not remember me by name, but . . . you baptized me in 1969. I was very sorry to hear of your illness . . . I would like so much to see you at Coral Hill again . . . I and everyone else are praying for you . . . Just remember that God is by your side ALWAYS. May God bless and comfort you.

Two friends recalled serious illnesses in their personal experience that had made lasting impressions on them. From Sierra Leone:

> Randy, the Lord used my illness of two years ago to help me reach new insights into our total dependence on His power, to see the value of prayer, and even pain and suffering. Of course, mine was not the length of your illness but I am

sure that His will is for you to pray for and expect His great power of healing.

From Colorado came this thoughtful letter:

I once knew a similar situation when faced with a diseased kidney . . . while it was tuberculosis, not cancer, those were times when medical expertise had fewer medicines and treatments than in those 1970s. I know how it feels to have your life suddenly altered, and I don't think I'll forget spending a complete year bed-fast, taking drugs daily. My own mother and father were told by doctors that my recovery was doubtful. Well, God obviously isn't necessarily limited by respectable medical opinion. Whatever else I may yet have to encounter, He answered my prayers and the prayers of others, and has spared me for times like these. It is this same loving God to whom I constantly talk in prayers about you. I believe with all my heart that He is able "to do exceedingly abundantly beyond all that we ask or think, according to the power that works within us," (Ephesians 3:20). The same God who showed mercy to me, Randy, can do more so to you if it is His will . . . the most consoling factor is the faith I have in Him who is able to comfort and keep you through His limitless love.

COVENANTS OF PRAYER

Many of the cards and letters, in fact most of them, revealed that people were participating in a covenant of regular daily prayer for me, my health, and my family. The firm belief in the God who answers prayer permeated these messages. At this point, I want to affirm that I have for a long time deeply believed in intercessory prayer. From biblical examples of God answering prayer to modern day examples, I've never doubted that power. I've also always believed that God is a healing God. He has the power, the love, and many times the will to specifically deliver people from physical sickness. I'm well aware that all prayer for healing and recovery does not result in every person's getting well. I believe that God knows all circumstances and answers in the way which, in His judgment, is best. Without a doubt, "all things work together for good to those who love the Lord . . ." but that does not mean that one who turns to God, in request for health, always receives it. Evil is a reality in our world; decay, sickness and death are a part of man's heritage as a result of sin.

I want to share a few notes indicating the nature of the prayer covenant into which so many entered for me. From Denton, Texas, a ladies' Bible class wrote:

> We are praying for you . . . May God grant you life and peace is our prayer.

From Denver:

> Our prayers for all of you are continuous. Remember the parable of the "importunate widow?" We are doing the same—asking God over and over and over. This we know—God loves you so much—and He is all powerful. Even as we are begging God over and over—so we are thanking Him over and over . . . please feel strengthened by ours (prayers).

From a dear lady:

> We love you, Randy, and continually lift you, Camilla, and the children into the Lord's hands; and I really trust Him to heal you.

From California, a college administrator speaking of the congregation of Christians where he worships:

> There is hardly a prayer where the entire congregation is involved that you are not mentioned by name. I promise you that we will continue to do that . . . We will also ask God to bless your wife and children during your temporary absence . . . We love you.

A couple from Abilene observed:

> People all over this town are crying out to the Lord for your total healing.

Another said:

> The Bible says "pray believing" and that's what a host of your friends are doing and we are among them.

From Oklahoma:

> Our prayers are for God's clearest interpretation to you of His purpose in this time of faith-building and development.

Although this "interpretation" is not yet totally clear, I am tremendously impressed with the ways in which God has brought good out of what appears to be only tragic. I'm thankful that during these months I have been privileged to see others' faith made stronger, their love grow deeper, their prayer life develop in fervor and other positive results of their having been touched by my experience. Even if my health falters in the near future, or if life here ends soon, I have really seen God's power to shine light into darkness!

Another letter, written by a beloved former teacher

of mine, who several years ago faced the uncertainty of cancer also, urged me in this way:

> We are all continuing to pray for you. I know that prayers by the thousands have been offered and I am sure that God will bless the chemotherapy which you are undergoing. I have found it a great comfort in my own crisis to pray earnestly and then leave the ultimate outcome in the Lord's hands. I know you have been doing that a long time

EXPRESSING CONCERN

If you have read to this point, you may be wondering how I really feel about the value of cards and letters to people who experience serious sickness. First, I must admit that without them my will to fight would have been diminished. My spirit wavered often, but I found genuine encouragement and felt the warmth of love repeatedly through cards and letters (as well as by phone and visits).

As for those who selected a card and simply signed their name, I was made aware that they were thinking of me. I was grateful. The personal expressions, such as those I have shared, and others, helped me know that I was enveloped in a real network of concern. From the young or the old, from the east or the west, from the sick or the well—from whomever, I realized the beauty of Christians' love for each other. How thankful I am that Jesus came and taught us how to love one another. He told his followers that the world would know him by his disciples' love for each other:

> By this all men will know that you are my disciples, if you have love for one another (John 13:35).

Some sent a card frequently, to brighten the day, to keep before me a physical reminder of their love. One particular family impressed me so much. Each member of the family wrote something personal on the note, mother, father, and four children. How beautiful to know that I was in the circle of that family's love.

I spoke to a group of college students recently and told them I hoped they would start a new movement—a movement to share their love and concern in situations like this by writing personal notes—selecting a favorite verse or thought—sharing a personal observation or experience—or in some way returning the personal touch to communications of concern. Beautiful cards are thoughtful, and as I said, I was grateful for every card that came with just a signature. That person thought enough of me to take the time to choose a card and send it to me. Still, I honestly must say that cards and letters that held personal expressions spoke so powerfully to me. Let me encourage you to think creatively of what you can share, in your own handwriting, to express your heartfelt thoughts to someone. I must emphasize that if a beautiful card and your signature best express your concern then by all means send that. Don't ever hesitate simply because you don't know what personal thing to say. Your signature says you care!

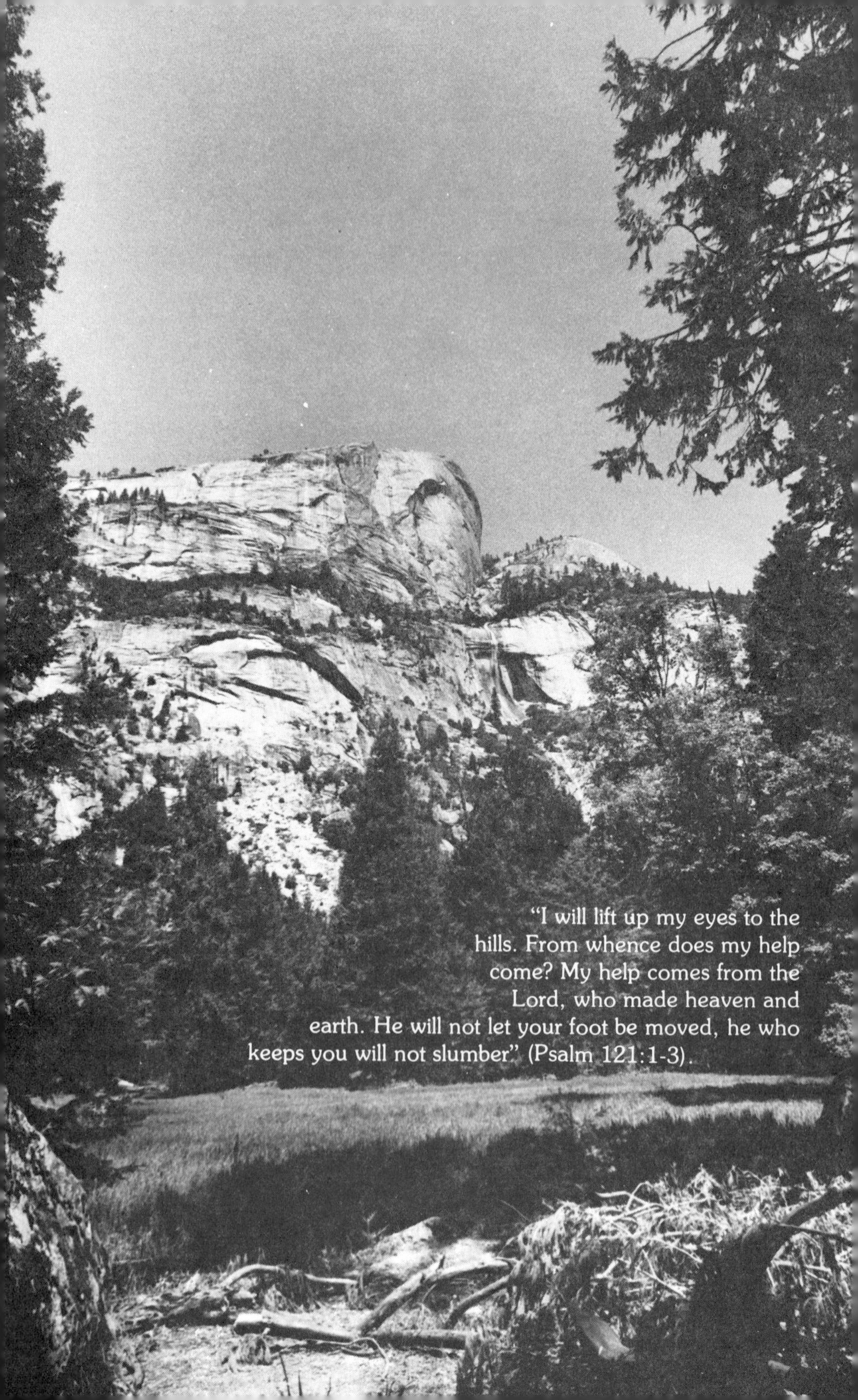
"I will lift up my eyes to the hills. From whence does my help come? My help comes from the Lord, who made heaven and earth. He will not let your foot be moved, he who keeps you will not slumber" (Psalm 121:1-3).

The Family of God

Once Jesus was speaking to the people when his mother and brothers came and wanted to speak to him. Scripture records this interesting response:

> But he replied to the man who told him, "Who is my mother, and who are my brothers?" And stretching out his hand toward his disciples, he said, "Here are my mother and my brothers! For whoever does the will of my Father in heaven is my brother, and sister, and mother" (Matthew 12:48-50).

The concept of the church being the "family of God" has always impressed me. The church is not a humanly devised organization; rather, it is people who have become brother and sister because of a new birth into the family of God. What brought us together? Redemption, God's mighty act of forgiveness through the death of His son. Every person who admits his need of God and responds obediently in faith is cleansed by trusting the blood of Jesus Christ for a right relationship to God. What do we have in common? We are now all God's children, members of His family, the church of Jesus Christ. This means to me that the Christian family is designed so that each of us takes total responsibility for the welfare of every other person. We're born of the same spirit, have the same Father, same Saviour, same work, same future.

THE FAMILY'S RESPONSE

How strengthening to my faith, then, was the way the church responded to my crisis. First, the crisis brought the family of God together in love, concern, and ministry to my needs. One congregation, with which I had periodically worked, immediately took up a special contribution to cover the financial expenses of Camilla and the children during the weeks in Houston. Women of another congregation supplied money for other related expenses of the Houston experience. My local congregation planned for a special contribution to help cover the enormous expenses of hospitalization and chemotherapy treatment. Individuals offered help if it were needed. Brethren blended their financial resources to meet the crisis.

Letters came revealing what was happening in the family of God.

> There has been such an awakening in our congregation of love and concern for you and your family . . . .

Another said:

> So many good things are happening here—and one of the most beautiful is how the concern of the family here for you has made us all feel closer to one another. It is a very expensive gift to give but it is one that you have given.

Another observed:

> Already here we are seeing evidences that love

> for each other is surfacing as we do what little we can to help you in your time of need.

And from another:

> I'm sure there are countless prayers being offered, even now, from people you have never met—I guess that is one of the great blessings of being in God's family . . . Our lives have been deeply touched . . . it has humbled us and brought us closer to our Father.

Not only by financial involvement, not only in a close-knit covenant of prayer, but also in personal commitment of time and ministry, the family reached out to me. There were those who served by looking after the needs of my family. Mothers took our children to play with theirs, freeing Camilla to spend time with me. Some Christian ladies found their way to help by looking after many of the responsibilities of my wife: housework, laundry, cooking. Some Christian men decided that whatever house repairs and work were needed would be their area of ministry. One brother came to the room, and stationed himself outside the door to meet those who came, giving them the latest report on my condition, thereby freeing my wife from that responsibility.

THE CHURCH'S MESSAGE TO THE WORLD

I've only mentioned a few ways in which the family of God reached out to support us in our time of need. There were many other individual acts of love and thoughtfulness in our situation. I firmly believe that the church speaks to the world when people see the church *being* the church, as in the actions I've described. The love shown to me was generated from God through the hearts of Christians. By this, I mean that every time we minister lovingly in the family, as well as to all men, we allow men to experience the love of God, to feel its warmth and to observe its transforming power. It gives us a foretaste of our home in heaven when we seek to fulfill each other's needs, either in time of crisis or simply in our everyday experiences. This is an expression of the genuine love we have one for another here.

When we truly love each other, we say to the world that we've experienced God's love and therefore we love one another, as well as those who are not yet in the family. By loving each other we are inviting the world to a love feast—God's love and the love of His children await each man who will come!

Life is a Gift

Watching newborn babies has always held quite a fascination for me. The wonder of life is experienced as we observe a person newly arrived into this world. From the first breath we become aware of the gift of life. Our environment, the air we breathe, the water we drink, the food we eat, all affirm the goodness of life. In reflecting on health I've noticed that many of us take it for granted, assuming our right to life; but have you thought very often of the early months and even years of your own life, when you were totally dependent upon others to assure that your life and growth would continue? As babies, we couldn't provide or plan for ourselves. It was out of our hands. Our life depended upon God's gifts. Those loving people who held us, loved us, and cared for our every need were gifts to us that we hadn't earned in any way.

Serious sickness has focused my attention once again on the wonder of life as a gift from God. If we consider life this way, we will keep fresh in our minds that every day must be lived fully, gratefully, because that day is a gift from God. One card I received displayed a beautiful sunrise and suggested, "Every sunrise is a message from God." That card is on a plaque in my office and sets the tone for my full appreciation of each day God gives. I don't believe man had a right to life, nor do I think that we can negotiate the length of our days.

"TODAY IS THE FIRST DAY . . ."

If you are like me, it may be that your life has been characterized by a perpetual "Looking Forward." See if you remember thinking this way:

> When seven years old—"I can't wait till I'm ten." When ten, "When will I be a teenager? They have all the fun!" At thirteen, "Oh, for my sixteenth birthday when I'll have a car." Sophomores in High School long to be seniors. Seniors look to graduation and college. College age looks to employment and independence that they feel comes with their degree. Then we look to marriage—then children, later we think of financial security, job accomplishment, then early retirement, and so it goes.

Now, I think a certain amount of forward looking is natural, healthy and to be expected. Yet many of us are aware that the forward look contributes to a de-emphasis of the importance of the day at hand. Although we are advised, "live one day at a time" we know very well that often on Mondays we anticipate the weekend eagerly. When you stop to realize that each day is a gift from God, you are able to slow down long enough to smell the roses, feel the wind, do the small kindnesses; in other words to live each day fully for its opportunities and delights.

I shall never forget the plane ride back from Houston after the long hospitalization. Having thought at times I might never see the outside world again, I was surprised when I was dismissed to find myself delighting in the sights, sounds, smells and people. Are we so busy that we no longer notice the beauty of God's world, the inestimable value of pausing long enough to notice the mysteries of life? I now find a great joy in looking at a tree, going to a park, seeing a sunrise, watching a child play; participating sensitively in the life experience; thanking God for each manifestation of His creativity, love, and provisions for His human family.

That's why I've come to feel that life's value and meaning will not be accurately measured by the number of years we live here, but rather by the way we live the years we are given. Quality life, abundant life does not require quantity life. Those who walk with God, having agreed with Jesus that their only will is to do His will, have found the key to abundant living. Walking with God allows me to maintain a stance of gratitude before Him for all His gifts.

FLOWERS WHILE THEY LIVE

I'm deeply touched every time I go to a funeral home. Usually there are numerous displays of flowers surrounding the departed one. They are given as an expression of love and concern. I've often wondered when I see those floral arrangements: "How many people sent flowers who did not, during the person's life, express their love in their relationship to the individual?" What a tragedy. I've always wanted my life to be characterized by the giving of flowers—the expression of love—to one while he lives. In other words, I wanted him to be able to smell the flowers now. This is another way to say:

I will pass this way but once.
If there is anything I can do

Let me do it now,
For I'll never pass this way again.

Is there anyone whose graveside service you'll attend with deep regret that your love was not expressed to the person while they lived here? I imagine we'll all have times like that, because we are weak. Still, wouldn't it be an affirmation of our desire to live abundantly if we committed ourselves to helping people smell the roses while they live!

Refocusing Life's Priorities

Rather than drifting through life, doing only those things at hand, I believe that we should all set priorities for our lives. We need to make commitments, invest our lives toward purposes that we can identify to be those of God. As a child of God I want to have His priorities first in my life.

For each of us, there are occasions when we re-evaluate our priorities. Some do this at the end of every year, others do it when major changes affect their lives. I did it while flat on my back. Out of re-evaluation can come new perspective, new understanding, new resolve.

One focus of my concentration on priorities was found in 2 Corinthians 5. In verse 15, Paul, speaking of Jesus, says:

> He died for all so that all who live—having received eternal life from him—might live no longer for themselves, to please themselves, but to spend their lives pleasing Christ who died and rose again for them (LB).

In verses 17-21 he describes what I believe to be the basic commitment of every Christian—that is, participation in God's ministry of reconciliation.

When someone becomes a Christian he becomes

> a brand new person inside. He is not the same any more. A new life has begun!
>
> All these new things are from God who brought us back to himself through what Christ Jesus did. And God has given us the privilege of urging everyone to come into His favor and be reconciled to Him.
>
> For God was in Christ, restoring the world to himself, no longer counting men's sins against them but blotting them out. This is the wonderful message he has given us to tell others.
>
> We are Christ's ambassadors. God is using us to speak to you: we beg you, as though Christ himself were here pleading with you, receive the love he offers you—be reconciled to God.
>
> For God took the sinless Christ and poured into him our sins. Then, in exchange, he poured God's goodness into us!

For me, this defines what my life work is. I'm privileged to participate in the very heart and nature of God by using my life—words and deeds—in the effort to bring men into the family of God. In other words, the first or top priority is people. People are important; things are not. I'm more aware now of the needs of people and find myself trying harder to spend the necessary time to help meet those needs.

THE MOST IMPORTANT PEOPLE OF ALL

An intensified commitment to people led me first to review my own family life. Nothing is more important to a husband and father than his wife and children. Although most men would agree to this, what really tops our list when it comes to our actual use of time? I believe it is a father's responsibility and privilege to introduce his children to God, by both his actions and his words. A child's first and most lasting impressions of God as his Father will usually come from his own father. I feel that a man makes a spiritual decision when he consecrates his family to God, committing that home to be a Christ-centered home.

In reviewing my family life I started by examining my typical weekday schedule. It went something like this: 8-5 work; 5-6 read the paper, watch the news; 6-6:30 supper; 6:30-7:30 miscellaneous, bathe the kids and put them to bed. It was startling to discover that my specified time with the children was less than one hour per day. That's not enough time for such an important relationship. Priorities had to be reordered. Paper reading, TV watching had to wait until later. From my arrival home until their bedtime the children would come first! What they want to play or to talk about now absorbs my attention and interest because they are very special to me and I want to be very special to them.

In talking with a successful businessman only a few days ago he told me of his wife's recent surgery for cancer. He said in a reflective moment, "You know, I really didn't know how sweet she was and how much I loved her until I thought about losing her." In my sickness, I have realized in a deep and meaningful way the tremendous beauty of my marital relationship. Words are totally inadequate here. The echo of an eight-year-old marriage vow, "for better or for worse, in sickness or in health" was a sustaining strength during cloudy days. The preciousness of a shared life and love is more real every day as a result of this experience. Walking through life with a loving mate means experiencing one of God's greatest gifts. To see love grow more mature through meeting adversity together is to better understand God's wisdom in creating the marriage bond. How difficult the days would have been without her by my side. Now, in these days, I am even more keenly aware than before of my opportunities to share happiness with her. Time together alone is so special. Time together as parents brings such joy. Time together in working toward common goals in God's service gives fulfillment. I have given such a small glimpse of the enormous importance of the husband-wife relationship, but perhaps enough to suggest that there is added depth and more radiant beauty now.

Doubts and Faith

The father of a child with a dumb spirit asked Jesus to help his son: "If you can do anything, have pity on us and help us (Mark 9:22). Jesus answered him: "All things are possible to him who believes" (verse 23). The father cried out, "I believe; help my unbelief" (verse 24). That father's anguished cry has been the prayer on many a Christian's lips during his pilgrimage of faith, including my own.

What is it like to believe and doubt? Is it wrong or natural to have periods of doubt in the Christian walk? Do we ever question God's love for us, especially when events and circumstances appear unfriendly to our welfare? Maybe you have identified with "doubting" Thomas who, after Jesus' resurrection, declared:

> Unless I see in his hands the print of the nails, and place my finger in the mark of the nails, and place my hand in his side, I will not believe (John 20:25).

The Bible describes our walk as Christians as walking "by faith and not by sight." Would you ever prefer to walk by sight? Maybe these questions are unimportant to you but they have become important to me. I raise them here for two reasons: first, I have experienced doubts during this illness and second, I have changed my thinking about doubts. Let me explain.

One of the first visitors that spent time with me during my initial hospitalization observed to another friend later that it seemed to him that I was afraid at that point in my experience. What struck him more than that, however, was that I seemed to be "afraid of being afraid." In other words, to this observer, I was upset because I was not calm and confident! Perhaps I expected too much immediately of my faith. Cancer is quite a shock. The announcement strikes a heavy blow at one's security base—good health. If his observation was correct, he may have sensed that I was a bit surprised that I could not simply face this jolt with quiet confidence and unquestioning faith. Afraid of being afraid? Maybe so. What strikes me in retrospect is that what I experienced was completely normal—an initial period of some fear and doubt. I'm not saying that all who face crisis go through this, nor am I necessarily saying it is good or bad. However, I do believe that some, perhaps many, face it.

Furthermore, the initial fear and doubt is not the only such experience. There are many periods of fear and doubt which threaten and/or strengthen one's faith in times of crisis. While expressing my times of doubt I have noticed two interesting reactions. First, there have been many friends, Christians, who choose to deny that I ever had any real or serious doubts. Perhaps momentary, they say, but not real or serious. Usually they base this denial upon their friendship with me and their belief that I have a strong faith. Unfortunately, these friends are incorrect. Secondly, there are those who suggest that only those who have really doubted are able to deeply believe. They accept the doubts as real and as a strengthening experience for faith. I appreciate both reactions.

BUT DOUBTS WILL COME

The fact is, doubts occurred. Not unlike Job's reaction when calamity struck, there is first a kind of numbed shock. Things looked utterly hopeless to Job at first. Then he felt anger and resentment. When Job talked with God about his dilemma, he became aware of some realities he had forgotten. God asked Job where he had been when the whole drama of creation had begun. God reminded Job of his good gifts, of the fact that all of Job's days had come from the same source. After Job's encounter with the Ultimate One Himself, Job had a new perspective on the past and a new vision of the future. I agree with Myron Madden, who wrote "the essence of despair is relegating God solely to the past." Job learned that he still had a future in God, for God had a future for Job.

The calamities of life are all deeply mysterious. It seems the more we try to "explain" them to each other and fix the blame and responsibility here or there, the further we get from the truth. What matters is the nature of life itself, and the One Who gives it.

One reason I mention Job is because a basic question that comes up is the "why?" of a crisis such as I experienced. I believe the answer lies in the nature of evil and its effect on our lives. However, after every possible "why" is considered and is found to be just that—"possible"—we are left to make a decision about whether we choose to trust or choose not to trust.

One of the immediate doubts is whether God really loves you. If He does, why would He allow disease to strike you down? If He does, then surely you will get well and not die. These thoughts entered my mind and would not leave. How did I handle them? Not easily, I assure you. First, I really thought seriously about God's love. Had He not always taken care of me? Didn't I have years of evidence of His loving care? The answer was yes. Still, the past was not in question. Today was my concern. I remembered that Paul in Romans 8 said that nothing could separate me from the love of God in Christ Jesus. Did that include cancer? My doubts were best handled by a conscious decision to trust. Trust can be given to one who has proven trustworthy. Every time I thought of the cross of Jesus I realized that my salvation was secure, that although my walk here might be temporary, my eternal walk with God had been permanently assured by Jesus Christ my Lord. Every time I wondered if I could trust the future to Him I remembered what a good job he had done with the past.

How natural it is when you are in a tunnel to want to see the light at the end. Who willingly trades the known for the unknown without any apprehension? "Now faith is the assurance of things hoped for, the conviction of things not seen" (Hebrews 11:1). Do I have faith? Yes. I decided once and for all into whose hands I would entrust my life when I became a Christian. I reaffirm that decision every day, when times appear good and when they do not; but doubts occur. When they do they present fresh opportunities for self-evaluation and a recommitment to faith in God. That is why the prayer is appropriate: "I believe, Lord; help my unbelief."

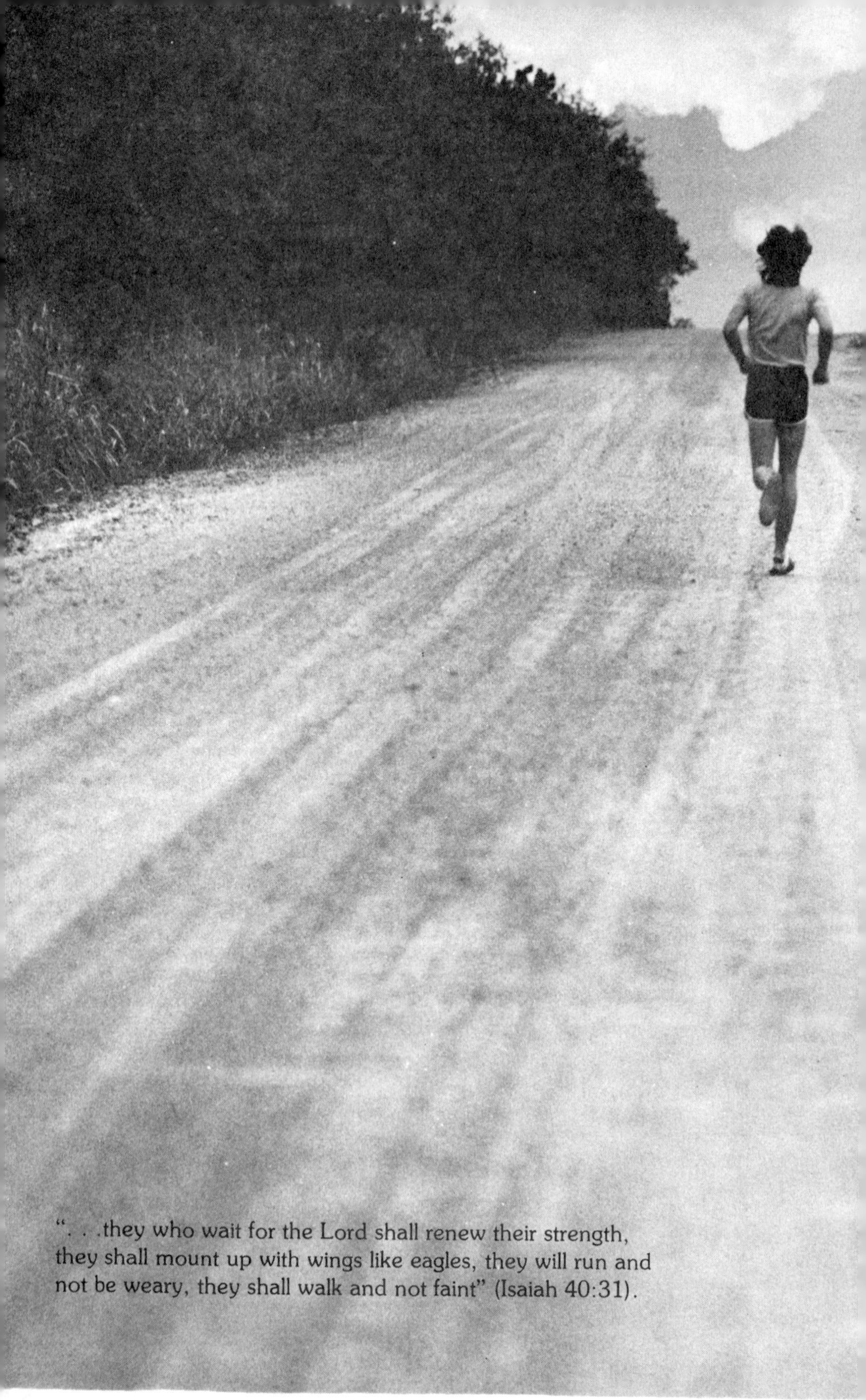

". . .they who wait for the Lord shall renew their strength, they shall mount up with wings like eagles, they will run and not be weary, they shall walk and not faint" (Isaiah 40:31).

The Meaning of Servanthood

In Mark 9 Jesus asked his followers, as they came to Capernaum, what their conversation had been about while on the road. Their response was an embarrassed silence; they had been discussing with one another which of them was the greatest. He called them to him and said:

> If anyone would be first, he must be last of all and servant of all." And he took a child, and put him in the midst of them; and taking him in his arms, he said to them, "Whoever receives one such child in my name receives me; and whoever receives me, receives not me but Him who sent me (Mark 9:35-37).

On another occasion James and John requested special places of honor when Jesus came into His glory. When the other disciples became indignant at the presumption of these two ambitious ones, Jesus said to all of them:

> You know that those who are supposed to rule over the Gentiles lord it over them, and their great men exercise authority over them. But it shall not be so among you; but whoever would be great among you must be your servant, and whoever would be first among you must be slave of all. For the Son of man also came

> not to be served but to serve, and to give his life as a ransom for many (Mark 10:42-45).

When Jesus used the object lesson of the child, he was saying something about the real values of human life. In contrast to their arguments about prestige, power and precedence, he talked about the child's spirit. Although not all children demonstrate it, the ideal child spirit is one of willingness to learn because he does not know, of willingness to trust. Children rarely have hidden motives or ambitions; they are aware of the wonder in God's world.

When replying to James and John's request, Jesus told the group that the goal of the follower of God is not to be a ruler, but rather to be a servant. Self-seeking is a common worldly value but Jesus turned this worldly value upside down by demonstrating, through his own life, the meaning of servanthood. The world will never recover from the impact of the Son of God deliberately taking upon himself the role of a servant when he walked the earth. The giving of his life as a ransom for man was the ultimate demonstration of his servanthood. From the cross all Christians find their model, their inspiration and motivation to lay down their lives in selfless service. The truly revolutionary nature of Christian fellowship lies in Jesus' servanthood. If you are like me you find it difficult to grasp the call of God to be a servant. Maybe, like me, you would say that you have not seen many models of servanthood in your life. You may even wonder why I brought the subject up in the first place.

There are three reasons why I am sharing my thinking about servanthood. In my sickness, I saw more clearly than I had ever seen before that God has called each Christian to be a servant—that within this concept lies the central meaning of living a Christian life. Second, I have seen some real servants during this experience, one in particular that I want to describe to you. Third, one of my most fervent desires, in the time God gives me on earth, is to learn how to be a servant. Thank God, He is teaching me. Maybe it took such a definite experience for me to gain a glimpse of what it means. I am not sure I can communicate my meaning but it is certainly worth the effort.

Before I describe in modern-day terms what it means to be a servant of the Lord, there is one other passage that will serve well as further background. In John 13:1-20, Jesus sat at supper with his disciples shortly before he was to be betrayed. It was a significant and moving time when fellowship was meaningful for he knew what lay ahead for him. He poured water and began to wash his disciples' feet. Scripture says they didn't understand why he did this. After washing their feet he said to them:

> Do you know what I have done to you? You call me Teacher and Lord; and you are right, for so I am. If I then, your Lord and Teacher, have washed your feet, you also ought to wash one another's feet. For I have given you an example, that you also should do as I have done to you. Truly, truly, I say to you, a servant is not greater than his master; nor is he who is sent greater than he who sent him. If you know these things, blessed are you if you do them (John 13:12-17)

What did Jesus want the disciples to know, to feel, to do? He wanted their commitment to walk as a servant as he had walked as a servant. Every time they thought of the Lord they would remember a servant. Every time they reflected on a "teaching" from the teacher, they would remember that he taught them the meaning of servanthood.

HOW CAN I BE A SERVANT?

Now, reflecting on these passages, what is required of one to be Jesus' servant? It seems that one must first understand who is the Lord of our life—that is Jesus Christ. He is Lord because of who he is (God's son) and what he has done for us (saved us from our sins). He has the absolute right to direct our lives. Until you and I make a decision about who will control our lives we will have no interest in being a servant. We either serve ourselves, which is called serving sin in the Bible (Romans 6:6-13), or we choose to surrender our lives to Jesus as our Lord.

Once we have made a decision about the cross of Christ—our salvation—we are then ready to "take up our cross and follow him"; in other words, to let him show us His way of life. Although I believe we spend a lifetime learning how to walk the Christian life, we begin with a heart that seeks to understand how to be a servant.

How does God teach us to be servants? First, he prepared a perfect human pattern for us so that we would not be at a loss to understand servanthood—the life of Jesus. He really is our example. It is a misconception to think one cannot follow in Jesus' footsteps. Surely, we can. Without ever stumbling? No, we'll stumble often, but we'll also succeed. Why? Because God has promised to help His children learn to walk like Jesus. That's the thrill of Christian growth. That's why I identify with the one who, when others seemed frustrated over his repeated mistakes, said, "Be patient, God is not finished with me yet."

So the pattern is Jesus. Second, the power is in God's Word and Spirit. We are led by the spirit of Christ as we learn to be servants through the study of God's Word.

Now, to the key point I want to make: there really are modern-day servants of Jesus Christ. It is one thing to know you have been called to be a servant, and that Jesus was a servant, but most of us really wonder: are there any servants around so that we can see what the life-style is like? The answer is yes. This doesn't mean there are any that are perfect servants; it simply means there are some in whose lives one can see clear evidence of their commitment to be servants of Jesus Christ. Further, it means that my life can be re-examined in light of their examples of servanthood.

A LIVING EXAMPLE

In my crisis, one particular servant, Landon B. Saunders, helped me see the true meaning of being a servant. Although we had been friends and co-workers before the crisis, I was never so aware of his servanthood as when it was directed toward me. First, he placed the highest priority on the needs of another person. His personal schedule, personal finances, personal conveniences were all adjusted so that he could be in the best position to serve me in whatever way he could.

The apostle John said:

By this we know love, that he laid down his

> life for us; and we ought to lay down our lives for the brethren (1 John 3:16).

Laying down one's life for another requires complete selflessness; inspiration for such selflessness is found in Jesus' laying down of his life for you and me. Servanthood calls for me to see the preciousness of a man's life over all else, to love as God loves and to give up myself in whatever way is needed to meet another's needs.

Landon accepted me just as I was through this experience. When I was lonely, or frightened, or doubting, or faithless, or brave, or callous, he always affirmed my personal worth. God's servant will accept people where they are and love them for what they are. He loved whether I was lovable or not. He sought to understand this experience from my perspective, to identify with my feelings. Yet, more than simply empathizing, he sought to bring the loving correction of God's truth, His will, into my heart at every opportunity. God's servant helps people face reality, helps them see God's way to face life and death. He sought to stand on the rock foundation of trust in Jesus Christ and to help me stand on it, when it appeared that all around was sinking sand.

His liability for me was total. He didn't worry about protecting his emotions, keeping emotional involvement at arms' length. He got involved, totally, and risked the possibility of getting hurt. He was completely willing to experience with me the "valley of the shadow of death."

Some specifics of his servanthood stay with me. Like the nights that were so lonely when he would simply sit in the corner of the room and wait until sleep finally overtook me. What thoughtfulness to be willing, without request, to share troubled nights in silence by giving one's presence to combat the numbing loneliness.

What servanthood to count it no sacrifice to cancel a schedule or rearrange one's commitments because a human being is in need. Didn't Jesus do that all the time? Was anyone unworthy of his concerned attention?

Landon's servanthood had no financial limitations. Personal debts were likely, in the prolonged hours spent in the hospital, but no importance was placed on the financial cost of his involvement.

I remember clearly many hours of conversation, especially when the valleys of depression were so overwhelming. How this must have drained him emotionally and challenged him spiritually! Yet he never wavered; he always hung in there, tough in the fight for me to have a healthy spirit and a vibrant faith.

During these months of treatment, we have had a precious prayer covenant, whether together or apart, about God's will and purpose in this experience. His love is continually demonstrated by his attention to my needs, whether physical or spiritual.

Have I described a modern-day servant of Jesus Christ and fellow men? What impresses me most, perhaps, is that this kind of servanthood characterizes Landon in his daily walk with other people also. I tell about our relationship as an example of servanthood, not so that anyone will think more highly of Landon than he ought or give him praise and honor, but so that you and I can think about the beautiful way in which God works through a yielded life, a life that desires to be a servant. Only God is to be glorified for Landon and servanthood. Jesus Christ and his way are understood by us more clearly because of the way in which Landon allows Jesus to live in him, directing his relationships with people. I want to be like him because he is like Jesus. I believe God will help me be a servant of men just as he helps Landon, and as he helps each one who brings a heart desirous of service.

Was Landon the only example of servanthood I saw? No, only the closest. There were many and each one is precious to me and is cherished. In fact, several demonstrated characteristics that I have tried to point out in Landon's life.

Visiting the Sick

These thoughts are the basic notes of a speech given to a group of preachers in Houston recently. Admittedly they are only reflections on my own hospital stays and are not meant to be hard and fast rules. One should only test these thoughts against his own study and experience to glean what is useful.

Visiting the sick has the potential of being a great ministry. However, it requires sensitivity, spiritual preparation, and good judgment if it is to be for the glory of God. I share these thoughts from the viewpoint of one who has been seriously ill on more than one occasion, and also from the viewpoint of one who has tried to be of service to those who are sick. The following observations are intended to encourage and help those who seek to minister to the physically ill.

When is the best time to visit? Generally, hospital patients need little if any visitation. Especially is this true with serious illness. One should ask: what motivates me to want to visit? Usually the answer is that one wishes to express love and concern in some physical way to the sick person. Sometimes we overlook several key considerations, however, if the goal is to show love and concern, could it be that other acts could do this better than a visit? My own experience has shown several ways.

One Christian decided to look after the physical needs of my family, never coming to see me but showing how very much he loved me by looking after my loved ones. Some Christian ladies found their way to help by looking after all the needs at home for my wife. Some mothers sought to keep my children with theirs in order to lighten my wife's load, freeing her to spend more time with me. Some Christian men decided that whatever house repairs and work were needed would be done. Others regularly found the time to give some cheerful item, card, flower, etc. as an expression of love. Still others found their ministry in the giving of money to help defray expenses.

When considering a hospital or home visit, generally it is most helpful to go only on the condition that the one sick wants visitors. Sometimes it is hard to know for sure; the safe way to know is by waiting two or three days after surgery and by checking with the family or close friends to see how well the patient feels. It is a good practice to bluntly ask a knowledgeable person if a visit would be desired.

Another condition is to go only when you are prepared to contribute toward recovery. If each visit does not contribute to the patient's recovery, it may have done harm rather than good. Are you willing to stay only a few moments? If not, you are not ready to visit. Do you have some encouragement? Can you be a good listener? Can you stay if you see you are needed? If not, maybe you should help in another way, rather than a visit.

What should be done in a hospital or home visit? Referring again to serious sickness, a patient should be helped, uplifted, inspired through a visit. Your presence should brighten the spirit, making the patient's state of mind better than before the visit. There are no set formulas for the content of a successful visit, but I found the following observations true in my own case. I wanted people who knew the Lord Jesus to come and visit me. I wanted people who knew what it means to hurt, having experienced disappointment or pain, and who knew how to empathize with my situation. I didn't want pity, but understanding and acceptance. I wanted them to hurt with me, to be one with me. I wanted a visit to refresh me from the monotony of the hospital room and the hours of being bedfast, even at home. I wanted someone who would share something from the outside world with me, something good that was happening. When visiting, be sensitive in conversation. What you have to talk about may or may not be the best therapy for the patient. Ask yourself: whom does this conversation interest, me or the patient?

When reading the Bible to someone, only read what you believe would be especially meaningful. Choose parts of the Bible that bring God closer, that tell us how much He cares. It may be that the patient wants favorite verses read to him; if so, do it. Otherwise, bring him a powerful pointed message through what you read. Remember, too, there may be times when he doesn't want the Bible read. Again, think of the patient's desires, not your own.

How long should I stay? Most of the time ten minutes is sufficient for visiting a sick person. If it is obvious the patient doesn't feel well then one should leave very quickly. In fact, a written note laid on a nightstand to be read later may be the most effective visit at some times. However, if a patient pleads for you to stay, it is a blessing for you to stay for a while. Presence is powerful when requested. There is a sense of identity in facing the crisis together.

What about prayer? Contrary to popular belief there are appropriate and inappropriate times for prayer. Be sensitive. Be sure the patient wants to pray; he may be in such spiritual or physical turmoil that he feels any prayer from him would be hollow. If this is the case your prayer will be for your benefit, not for the patient. If he is experiencing doubt or anger against God, you may want to pray for him, but it would probably be best to do so privately. Don't push the patient. If you pray with him, make your prayer relevant and sensitive to the illness and perspective of the sick person. For example: avoid being too simple when talking of pain, for there is nothing worse than lightly regarding pain. Of course, don't overplay pain, for no one wants pity, only understanding. Try to be understanding when you pray. Pray for God to directly intervene. Call upon Him for lessening of pain, quickness of recovery, endurance in suffering. Pray believing. The patient needs to know you believe in God's power and willingness to heal in order to lift his spirit.

These thoughts are only a beginning. They are shared to encourage intelligent, thoughtful visiting of those who are ill.

Reflections from A Fellow Struggler

Periodically I go to Houston for tests and checkups, often spending many hours in the outpatient clinic with as many as 1,000 others. As I read, meditate, and watch these people I have a deep empathy for them. I often think about whether or not they have a relationship with God. Do they have eternal hope, regardless of the outcome of their disease? I've wished I could sit and visit with each, sharing the good news of our Saviour. Upon returning home recently I wrote down some thoughts about what I would say if I could visit individually with each. This contains some of the ideas that I would use if I could visit personally at length with someone.

I have been coming to M. D. Anderson Hospital for about one year now. I have lymphosarcoma, cancer of the lymph system. The treatment here reflects the best in cancer research in our nation and the personnel are characterized by professional competence and personal concern. If you are like me you are grateful to be able to come here with your health problem.

Also, you probably realize the seriousness of cancer and have found time for careful reflection on the meaning of your life. I have. Having been hospitalized here and then having had an extended period as an outpatient in the clinic, I have found that there is much time for thinking. Let me briefly share with you.

One of my most frequent reflections is that life is a gift from God. From early childhood each of us has observed that life has an end; that in fact, everyone is terminal. What is important, then, is that life be lived to the fullest; each day must be enjoyed for the gift that it is. Quantity of days is not so important as is the quality.

I have observed that each of us is primarily interested in three questions about ourselves—who we are, why we are here, and where we are going. I have thought about those questions frequently. May I share with you briefly some answers that have given me meaning for life?

Who am I? I am a unique and important creation of God. He created me to live, to love, to give Him glory through my life. We are all God's children, living in His gift to us: the world. Unfortunately, because of man's rejection of God's authority and his bid for independence a long time ago, many of us are now confused about who we are. We have either forgotten we are His children or we have rejected Him as our Father. We are made in God's image. We are definitely His and that is why it is such good news that He loves us very much. A very appealing verse shows us how much He loves us:

> For God so loved the world that He gave His only Son that whoever believed in Him might not perish but have eternal life (John 3:16).

He loves you and me so much that Jesus' death on a cross took place so that we could be given life that will not end.

Why am I here? On the wall in my home is a plaque that states:

> I shall pass this way but once.
> Therefore any good that I can do
> Or any kindness that I can show
> Let me do it now
> For I shall not pass this way again.

I am here to honor God with my life. He is honored by my loving Him with all my heart and loving my neighbor as myself. A tall order, you say? Yes, the challenge of a lifetime, but the highest calling a man could have. The fulfillment and happiness of a life of service is lasting. Jesus was a servant of men, ultimately performing the greatest service—laying down his life for you and me. Even with all the hypocrisy we see around us every day, there is still nothing more beautiful than someone honestly attempting to live as a simple Christian. The service and love which flows from one Christian genuinely brightens this world in which we live.

Where am I going? Life here is brief, at best. Someone has described it as a vapor that appears for a little while and then is gone. Yet man, God's unique creation whom he loves and cares for, has a future. It is a future only with God. All of us will walk through the valley of the shadow of death, as Psalm 23 tells us. Is there anything worse than being totally alone when facing life's grand finale? My confidence is that I will not experience that step into the unknown alone. When I walk the valley, God's hand will reach out and clasp mine and lead me to that eternal home He has prepared especially for all men who respond to His love.

This leads me to ask you, a fellow traveler in this way of life: what are your personal answers to these questions that I have reflected briefly on: Who am I? Why am I here? Where am I going?

I know you have thought about it. Maybe you want to think more about it. If I were able to talk personally to you it would be so meaningful. Since I cannot I simply wanted to share these reflections.

One final thought: when faced with the crisis of life, such as the cancer experience, one needs to know something secure, someone who can be trusted, something to give us more than temporary hope. Many of us may, with excellent medical help and God's grace, overcome this disease totally, or at least be long-term survivors. Some of us will not. I have decided to trust God and, whether I live or die, commit my life to Him. Why? He made me, has cared for me through the years, has forgiven me my rebellion against Him and invited me to be His friend through my acceptance of His love. He has promised eternal life to those who admit they are not self-sufficient, to those who choose to put Him first in their lives. I invite you to do the same. It has given me peace, love, purpose and hope.

I close these reflections with two personal requests. One, if you would like to correspond with me about your answers to life's questions or if you want to really consider becoming a simple Christian, without denominational affiliation, please do. Second, maybe the problem of human suffering and disease is a real mystery for you and you would like to consider how

God relates to this problem. I have thought about this often and would like to share a printed consideration of it with you.

Now, what are the obligations? None. In fact, if you choose to remain anonymous when you write, that is all right. My only motive is to share. There is no hard-sell follow-up of any kind. The fact that you read this is gratifying to me. By the way, if you have cancer I want you to know I feel very close to you and urge you to live each day fully and keep up the fight.

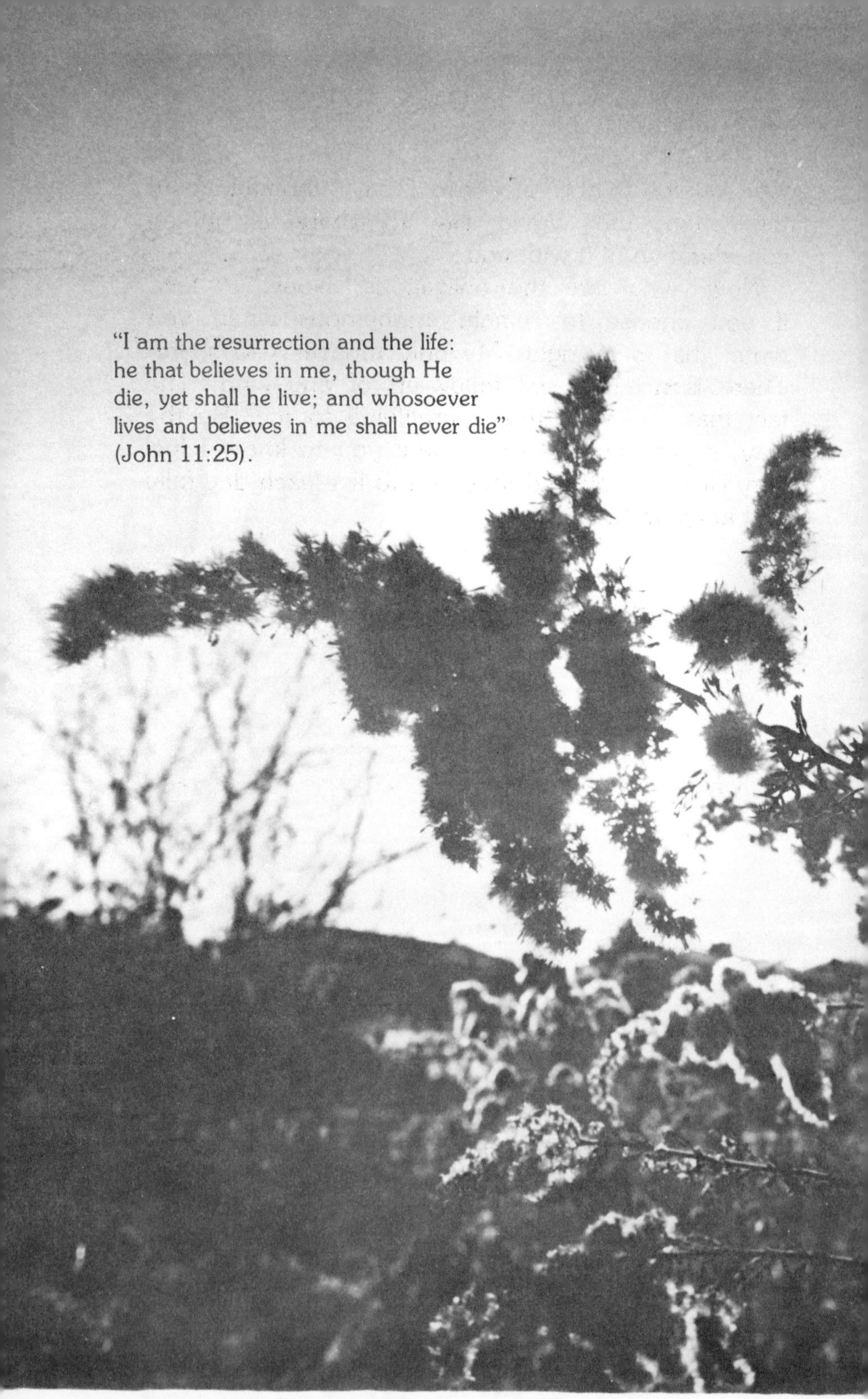
"I am the resurrection and the life: he that believes in me, though He die, yet shall he live; and whosoever lives and believes in me shall never die" (John 11:25).

"That the Son of Man May Be Glorified"

On July 2, 1974, nine months after my original diagnosis, I was privileged to speak to an evening worship service at the Highland Church of Christ. I deeply love this church where I have been a member for several years. The love of this church for me and my family was a tremendous blessing during these times. The following is the edited transcript of that message.

From John 11:1-4:

> Now a certain man was ill, Lazarus of Bethany, the village of Mary and her sister Martha. It was Mary who annointed the Lord with ointment and wiped his feet with her hair, whose brother Lazarus was ill. So the sisters sent to him, saying, "Lord, he whom you love is ill." But when Jesus heard it he said, 'This illness is not unto death; it is for the glory of God, so that the Son of God may be glorified by means of it."

Most of you know the rest of the story of Lazarus. It has impressed me during the last eight months of my own illness that Lazarus' illness is referred to as being "for the glory of God."

My prayer and many of your prayers have been that somehow out of my own illness God could be glorified. For we're all but a vapor, as James says; we appear for a little while and then we're gone. And it seems that the goal of each of our lives is to glorify God, whether that be by health or by illness, by life or by death. It's hard for us to learn that the gospel tells us that whether we live or whether we die we are the Lord's. Everything's all right, because he has claimed our lives. His death on the cross made all that happens to us have meaning. I don't know how people endure serious illness without faith in God. Serious illness teaches so many things about this world—about our value system, about the things that we treasure and hold dear. Without faith in God one's life is shattered by illness.

Tonight, I want to do something a little bit unusual in this lesson: give you a progress report on my personal health. That's an awfully personal thing to do, but many of you have been praying, fervently, regularly, daily, that God would heal me. God has answered that prayer and is continuing to answer it. I hope that there is no Christian here who does not have a deep realization of the power of prayer. When we call upon the Father, He hears and He answers. That ought to shake us to the very foundation of our being. We are so significant in the sight of the God who made us that he hears us and answers when we pray.

Last Tuesday, I spent another day waiting for a doctor in Houston to tell me what the next round of my treatment would be. I've been taking treatments once every two weeks for the last eight months. In November, when I first became sick, many of us didn't really know how sick I was; I was the least informed of all. I think from that point to this, there's been a great story. It's a story, not about me because I'm something, but about the power and the grace of God.

People went to the throne of God immediately and asked Him for His will to be done—but if it could be His will, that this illness would end in a restoration to health.

Last Tuesday, my doctor told me that I'm in complete remission now. Now for anyone who has cancer that's tremendously good news; that's the goal of all the treatment. Just so that we're clear about what God has done and what could lie ahead, I should tell you that at present there's no cure for what I have. They don't talk about cure for certain kinds of cancer—they talk about remission. This means that this growth stops, that it is surrounded by good healthy tissue, that there will be no ill effects on my life because of this cancer. So from the first day of my illness those who know me and love me have been praying for remission, and that's precisely what has happened, by the grace of God. I believe that He would not have done so had He not been asked by those who love me, many of whom are in this church.

So it's deeply moving to me to know that I've been the object of that kind of praying, and that I've been the battleground on which the grace of God has been fighting, and is victorious. I think there's a cause for great thanksgiving. I think it's an occasion for great thanksgiving whenever we ask God in faith and He answers as He has done in my life. Regardless of whether this goes out of remission, which it could do at any time, regardless of what happens in the future, God has done a great deed to this date. He spared me, and I think it's for a work. I told someone the other day I thought God was preparing me for something—I wasn't sure what it was.

I think He has been at work in my life through this illness, and I'm beginning to get a glimpse of what I think is the purpose. I think that it is so that through my life souls can be won, that people can be moved toward God, whether I live a short time or a long time. Each of us has only this day in which to live: none of us has any other days to count on. All of us ought to be able to say with the Psalmist:

> I love the Lord, Because he has heard
> my voice and my supplications.
> Because He inclined his ear to me,
> therefore I will call upon Him as
> long as I live (Psalm 116:1,2).

During my sickness, scripture meant a lot to me; people meant a lot to me. This church has meant a great deal to me. We say that often, but very few of us have had the opportunity to have it demonstrated to us, as I have. This is indeed the family of God, and it's not too big and it's not too cold. It's warm and I think it's just the right size. (It just needs some growth.) I've been the object of love such as I've never seen before. I think the world has been looking for this kind of love, and has seen what Christian love is all about in the way that you have loved me. Many have been amazed that Christians are willing to do so much for someone they love.

It's been a lesson to me that if you love me so much, and you do, think of the love that we ought to be able to share with the world to bring them to Christ. I think the world is waiting to see that kind of love. Ought we not to show it toward one another so the world can see it, so the world can be brought to Jesus' feet?

There's another Psalm that means much to me, Psalm 30:2,3. I read it while in the hospital:

> O Lord my God, I cried to thee for help,
> and thou hast healed me.
> O Lord, thou hast brought up my soul
> from the grave,
> restored me to life from among those
> gone down to the Pit.

So many of the Psalms are from the heart of one who cries out to God for help. How it could cleanse our hearts of pride if we viewed ourselves as always being in need of God's help.

Illness, by its very nature, causes one to think about his own weakness. God's strength has always been seen most powerfully when man admits he is weak. I've seen the strength of God more as a sick man than I ever saw it as a healthy person. I don't wish illness on anyone, but I do pray that every time illness comes we can do several things. First of all, use the time to reaffirm the value of life; secondly, call to God, who is the giver of life for the restoration of health; and thirdly, praise His name when it comes.

Now we have appendectomies and a sore nose and broken arms all the time. We just expect them to get well. We're not as grateful as we ought to be even when we're healed of those things; but when God gives us health, among His other gifts, we ought to thank Him and praise His name. Health is to be treasured as a gift of God. I can say that because of my past experience, but you can believe it because you're enjoying health. You can thank God right now for the health you enjoy. You can dedicate it to His glory.

If you have your Bible I'd like for you to turn to Psalm 86. That Psalm often pulled me out of depression in the early days of my sickness. There's much in the Psalm that's so meaningful. I want to go back through it slowly and share with you what it has meant for me. I'm impressed first by the cry for God to incline his ear and answer, "for I am poor and needy." What does the Lord require of you? In the Old Testament we're told one of the treasures God wishes you to lay on the altar is a contrite heart. We can be made in the image of Christ only as our hearts are able to be molded, only as God can reach us, only as we admit our need for Him. The Psalm starts off

> for I am poor and needy . . .
> Thou art my God; be gracious to me, O Lord,
>   for to thee do I cry all the day.
> Gladden the soul of thy servant,
>   for to thee, O Lord, do I lift up my soul.

Notice what he says next: "For thou, O Lord, art good and forgiving, abounding in steadfast love to all who call on thee." Do you ever tire of praising God? Now be honest. Man was formed for the purpose of giving praise to God. I wonder if we tire of praising Him. Can you exhaust His goodness descriptively as you pray? I don't think we can, and I don't think I spend enough time praising Him. We've decided not to praise God too much; we don't want someone to think we're emotional, so we limit our emotions as we praise God. Yet I hear the Psalmist here crying out in describing God's goodness and His loving kindness and His willingness to forgive. As God gives you and me days, I hope that we can praise His name every day. I pray that's the tone of your prayer life, and that's the tone of what you talk to your children about—the goodness of God. How much we take God for granted! I've been among the foremost offenders. God has richly blessed you, so remember to praise His name.

Someone said to me as I shared the report of how good the remission is at this point, "Don't forget to thank God, because it'll be a great sin if you don't." I have thought about that often. How many times we pray for things and forget to thank God when they come our way; The ingrate is among the most hated of people, particularly when we are the ones who did the favor. Children or friends or strangers—whoever —the ungrateful hand is a cursed hand. Yet, how often we're ungrateful to God for what He's done for us.

> Give ear, O Lord, to my prayer;
> hearken to my cry for supplication.
> In the day of my trouble I call on thee,
> for thou dost answer me.

I've learned never to be ashamed to call upon God in time of need. Some people call that a crutch. If so, then thank God for that crutch! I just wonder if we ought to call upon God more. Realizing the trouble that we live through and the fears that we have, we need to pray when we're afraid or in trouble. That's a golden time to pray because God is strong and we're weak. Oh, that we would call on Him in the good times; but, oh, let's call on Him in the troublesome times because He's there and He hears!

Then the Psalmist turns in verse 11 to the request

Teach me thy way, O Lord,
  that I may walk in thy truth;
Unite my heart to fear thy name.

I wonder how honest I've been sometimes when I've asked God to teach me. He longs to teach me His Word, but how often I keep His Word closed, and He can't reach me! If you really long to know the will of God you want to have it written on your heart. You must give God the opportunity to write it there—through the study of His Word. The Bible has come to mean so much, daily, to me. The Word is truly a lamp and a light unto our way, but we can't be taught if the word remains shut except on Sundays and Wednesdays. "Teach me thy way, O Lord."

I've had time to reflect not only on these Psalms, but also on the church. This church has meant so much to me. I've begun to understand what we mean when we say we need each other. Had I had to bear the financial burden without the help of Christians, I don't know what I would have done. It's expensive to be seriously sick; the bills continue to mount. Then, there was a day when you came together and gave generously in the special contribution to me. I thank you for it because you've united to fulfill a need that I couldn't have filled. I was helpless; God blessed me through brethren. I don't know what people do when they don't have that kind of support and love in time of need. I hope this means something to those of you who are healthy now. When sickness comes I want to pledge to you that this church will be there. I feel free to make that kind of pledge because this church was there for me, and this church continues to be there for me. When you're in need this church will envelope you in its arms and love you and take care of you. You ought to thank God for that, over and over; you ought to thank God for being a part of it. I thank God always for being a part of this kind of family.

What you've done for one of your own has been known as far east as Tennessee and North Carolina and as far west as Denver and Los Angeles. We tend naturally to do for our own, but it's good, it's loving, it's Christian. It makes an impression on us. I was embarrassed when I first heard of the contribution for me; I was frankly embarrassed that it was taken. I couldn't talk about it this freely had it not been for some letters I received while I was still in the hospital from Christians who were there during the service. These Christians said they had never been spiritually helped as much as in that service. If God could use that kind of service to strengthen or teach somebody what the family is about, then I can be gracious and thankful enough not to be embarrassed by it. There were letters that came saying "God is showing us something; we've never seen the unity of the church like we've seen it in the Highland church over your illness." Thank God for that unity Thank God for that kind of purpose. Thank God that tragedy can bring us together.

Today is a high point; today is a day for rejoicing; but there were low points and you walked in those low points with me. Thank God for the family. Now when we teach outsiders what the family of God is, this is what we're talking about. I'm a living example of what the family means and I intend to continue to teach that theme; I know you do too. It's beautiful to see it practiced. It's beautiful to see God doing things through His family. I've never felt stronger than I feel at this moment, and it's because of the grace of God. There have been prayers that I would even feel well enough to say what I have said tonight. If you ask me how I'm feeling, I will tell you that I feel tired all the time, but I feel good. I believe that God has in store a great deal of work for me and for you. He may call us home tomorrow, but I'm thankful that He's in control of that and we're not. He's heard prayer and He's answered. Now I want you to join with me in singing one verse of "How Great Thou Art."

I want to close my comments by asking you to continue to pray. There may be people who will say "Why pray now? God has answered, hasn't He?" But there's need for prayer, and I'm asking you to continue to pray because the story's not finished. God is to be petitioned further and regularly that His grace will continue to hold back this disease. That may sound like an awfully selfish thing, but there's no request that we ask of each other in the family that's really selfish. So I'm asking you to keep praying. You'll never know how much it means to me. People have been out of the country and said when they came back "I prayed for you every day I was gone." People have had burdens of their own but they've said "We pray for you every day." God is to be praised and I praise His name for that daily prayer.

Would you bow with me as we pray:

> Father I love You and each Christian here loves You. We love You because You're our Father. You've graced our lives by Jesus Christ and Your loving kindness, and Your grace has covered us and we feel your nearness and we want so much for our lives to be in harmony with Your

will. Would You, Father, take each life here that yearns tonight to be in Your will and draw them close and teach them Your way more perfectly? Would You take us, Father, as a family and help us to grow by adding brothers and sisters through the proclamation of Your gospel? As I devote my days to proclaiming Your will each of us devotes his days to proclaiming Your will. We devote ourselves to praising Your name for Your goodness. We're Your children; oh, how we need You, for without You we are nothing. We cry unto You, Father, because we're sinners, and we ask for cleansing, and we ask that our lives will be able to reach other people with the gospel. Make people look at us and see the way we live and come to You. This is our prayer, in Jesus' name. Amen.

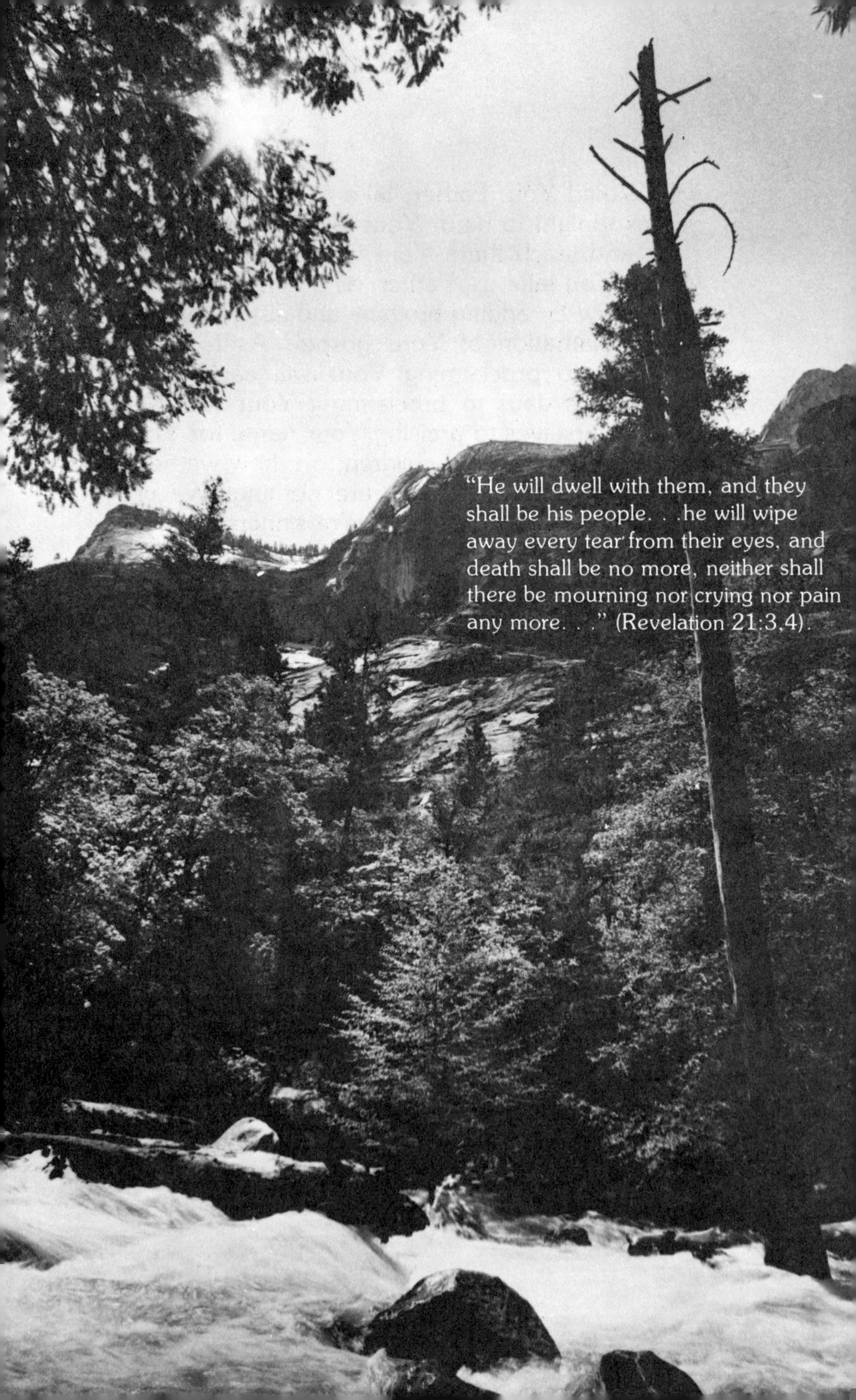
"He will dwell with them, and they shall be his people. . .he will wipe away every tear from their eyes, and death shall be no more, neither shall there be mourning nor crying nor pain any more. . ." (Revelation 21:3,4).

Conclusion

The first year of living with cancer is over. However, the impressions and lessons from this experience continue to unfold in my life.

However difficult these months have been, I choose to start the second year with faith and hope. The foundation for my faith and hope is God. In the midst of uncertainty, He is certain. And so, I continue my pilgrimage, walking hand in hand with God my Father.

“O Lord my God, I cried to thee for help, and thou hast healed me, O Lord, thou hast brought up my soul from Sheol, restored me to life from among those gone down to the Pit. Sing Praises to the Lord, O you His saints, and give thanks to his holy name. For His anger is but for a moment and His favor is for a lifetime. Weeping may tarry for the night, but joy comes with the morning. (Psalm 30:2-5).

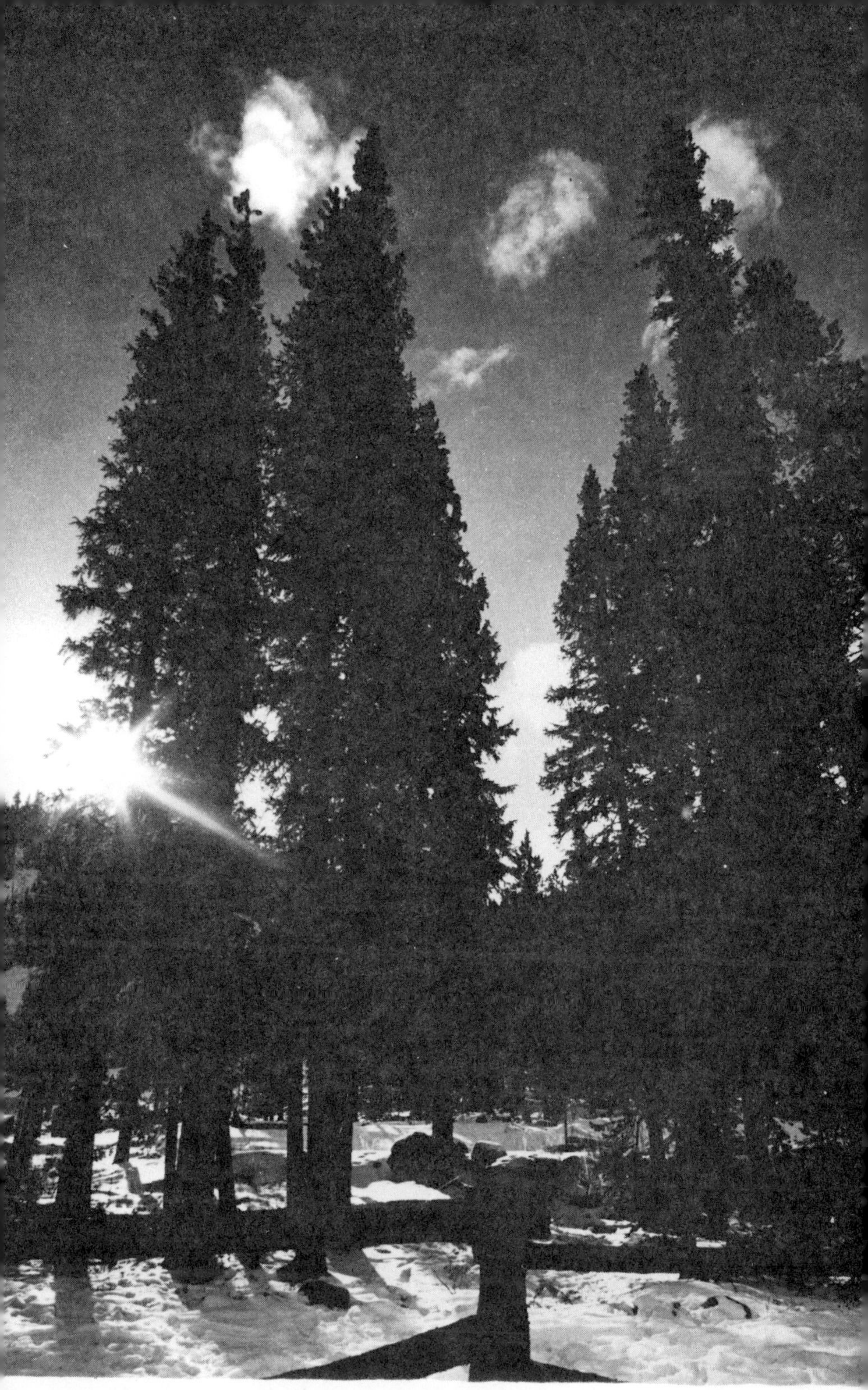